SHATTERED WINGS

I0563764

Marie Anne Zammit

chipmunkapublishing
the mental health publisher

Marie Anne Zammit

Published by
Chipmunkapublishing
PO Box 6872
Brentwood
Essex CM13 1ZT
United Kingdom

http://www.chipmunkapublishing.com

Edited by Marc Wilson

Chipmunkapublishing gratefully acknowledge the support of Arts Council England.

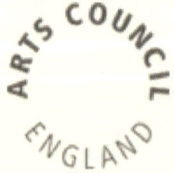

SHATTERED WINGS

DR. MICHELLE

Sex offender Report

I did it again, this time like in previous times, which brings me back again from where I started. These inner impulses seem like shadows walking alongside with me, or more like visions which never stop. These visions remain with me to give me pleasure and take me to heaven, and they keep coming like sweet dreams.

Are they dreams?

Yet, when I look back I say it was not really me who raped that young girl; but then who was it? Yes, it was me, and I did it and did it again. I can't help it; whenever I see a young woman, or even a girl, the fire starts burning deeply, tingling inside my head, until I do it. Then I find release.
And do I feel anything? Waves of ecstasy all over my body, and the more she resists the more pleasure I derive and feel transported into a world of bliss. This was my own world, my domain.
No one will understand this, but I do.

I do because it is in me, a deep surging thought residing inside me which cannot rest. In my thoughts I only see the girls resisting me, crying, and the more I force myself the more the ecstasy swarming all over me. This is not an invented story. It is the reality which haunts me day by day, and my sexual pleasure is only derived from that.

Well, I tried to do it normally, as it should be with other women; but doing it the proper way did not help. It was cold and mechanical and gave me nothing; not like when I do it with force. The pleasure attained when I assault a woman is different. It's my masterpiece, and twenty years locked behind walls are not sufficient to change me and stop me from raping.

I can still fantasise and conjure up images of rape, even during my time in prison. It helps me devise more enticing plan to seduce my girls. It would serve to kill time. Indeed, it serves as a vacuum for my dreams and nothing can change me as this is something which comes, no matter how hard I try. Do I try?

These impulses come as sweet showers of pleasure which taunt me, and they help me to erase all my troubles from my mind, and only fragments of one single memory remains, that of intense pleasure. Yet, my troubles commence when they deprive me of my dreams, and they have tried. In one of my first cases I was given a Probation Order for three years, hoping that I would stop, and so they put me on treatment.

It succeeded for a while, and perhaps my impulses slowed down; my fantasies decreased as well as my sexual urges. Well, I had no choice, and the only fantasy I was allowed to have was about my probation officer, a buxom woman with a pretty face. What else could I ask for? Thinking of her sends shivers all over my spine. Yet, she was hard as steel. I hate women who are hard. Women are made to be soft and supple so that we can taste their magic in their thighs. Oh what splendour when they moan and resist! I get even more excited.

The probation officer worked on controlling my beliefs and my impulses. She referred me to a psychiatrist, who gave me medication. This medication seemed to me like a cold shower to stop my warm dreams; they hate me and all they want is to stop me from visiting my secret place. That was not me, but another part of me which they wanted to get.

Three years under supervision was like hell to me. It is the revenge of the gods, for meddling with their nymphs. Yet, nymphs are soft and vulnerable, good to taste, and to feel their flesh is the ultimate. Every night I have this sensational dream of caressing the soft skin of a nymph, and then proceed on my journey. With the treatment I could do nothing. It suppressed me and blocked me from attaining my goal. It felt like a void and suddenly all the thrill and sensations derived from my exciting journey ebbed away.

I was stupefied and the thought was there but no action. Finally, it got on my nerves. I could not take it any longer but I had no choice. There was a Court Order and prison was no longer attractive. Prison is rather chilly, freezing my body and my thoughts where I only longed to taste the flesh of a nymph and to hear her crying while I forced myself deep inside her.

That was my conquest.

So, I waited impatiently, pretending that all was fine, and that I have changed my life, and that I had repented and changed my mode of living, away from the girls. I made them believe that. For two years I complied with them both, with the probation officer and the psychiatrist. They were pleased, and I told them what they want to hear. Little did they know about the dream which I had creating in the corners of my mind.

Two years of hell passed, like any thing in life, and the day of the termination of the order dawned. This day was special; I met the probation officer for the last time. I could well see the sensuality buried and put under control behind her tough, firm voice, and the muscles of her face taut, refusing to reveal any emotions. Yet I could easily detect her underlying message she avoided conveying. It was like a sixth sense, a subconscious feeling which overwhelmed me. She was a woman after all, but I did not dare.

The night came when I decided to let myself drown into the sea of my suppressed passions buried in the deep abyss of my desires. Joseph needed to be himself- the old passionate, ardent Joseph.

I waited for too long. The night was full of stars, promising a lovely journey of pleasure. After the restraints of the medication, my body was yearning forthe waves of passion. Spending two whole years without touching a woman are no joke. It is like starving for no reasonable purpose. I had waited far

SHATTERED WINGS

too long to taste the innocent sweetness of my angels. I was driving my car, embracing the new freedom which I have acquired. Then, I thought I was seeing an angel crossing my path. I stopped the car and asked her the time. She looked at me.
'It's 9.30 pm,' she replied.

I was not interested in the time, but in her pretty round face. An angel, soft and made just for me. Joseph, take action, be fast. I said to myself. Then it was time. I grabbed the girl and pushed her in my car. She was startled. Oh, little one if only she knew what was awaiting her! I locked the car and looked at her.
'Ok, my sweet,' I told her.
She looked terrified, and the more terror I see in their eyes the better. That means they will succumb. I was suddenly breathless and the pressure was already taking its toll. Two years on medication did not affect my performance, and that was pretty good news. Yet, the tormenting passion all over my body was overwhelming, and I could not wait to do it. Do it now, I thought.

So, I did it. I started with her breasts. They were soft and beautiful. In my hands they felt like silk. The little nymph tried to resist but there was no hope, no escape from me. I then headed for her thighs, soft as honey. I took a deep breath and started my voyage. For how many nights had I dreamt about this night? Countless! She was crying, but her sounds added to my excitement. The little voices of angels were begging me to act, so I went on to her lovely flower, as promising as her lips. She was soft as velvet and ripe as cherries. The nymph cried and cried, but I could not hear it. I only sensed her inner world. The more I forced myself, the higher I went, transported on waves of ecstasy. There, I felt I was living again. Joseph was born again, and he found his identity from raping nymphs.

Yes, I am a rapist, and no one can stop me. No court, no law can refrain my passions. I may stop for a while, but then I go back to my dream.

You still have to find ways to stop me from dreaming. Till then I will keep on raping, if not in reality, certainly in my dreams.

This is not fiction, but the thoughts of one of my patients, and these horrid lines were written by Joseph. My hands tremble as I hold the paper, but this is the reality of what besieged the mind of a rapist; a terrible, afflicting truth which at times we seek to evade and try to make ourselves believe it does not exist. They are around us and often closer to us than we can ever imagine. There were many like Joseph. Some controlled their thoughts and fantasies, others went further and committed crimes.

It was raining heavy all throughout the day and we were stuck in our office, so this gave me extra time to go through my reports. This report reflects the sheer reality of these particular patients, shocking words which are disturbing, but I have become immune and almost hardened by these facts. It occurs to me that we have failed with them, and they will one day take over us. Yet, the sullen looks of my patients coerce me to go on. The rain kept pouring and it seemed that it had done all day. Great, for at least it helps to alleviate us from the other days filled with heat and the fierce rays of the sun.

The yard at the mental hospital was deserted, abandoned by the usual residents who passed their time strolling about, at times chatting amongst themselves. That was their consolation, as if for one moment they came in tune with nature and left behind the thoughts which tormented them and their lives. It grieved me deeply to watch the deterioration of human beings, but that was life, and everything had to go with the flow of nature. And today it was a manifestation of nature. Yes, I thought as I watched the heavy drops slowly hitting against my window. This created a new sensation. I took a deep breath and then walked back to my desk. It's like entering back in the routine world. These were the thoughts as I waited; piles of files were standing on each other waiting for my attention. Yet, the job as a psychiatrist was most fulfilling.

My secretary, Angelle, entered my office. I looked at her and noticed that there was something different. Then it occurred to me that it was her hair. Today it was bunched up neatly, not the usual waves hanging to her shoulders. She was pretty, with dark hair and dark skin, but best of all Angelle was always focused on her job. However, there were times when I thought she was wasting her time in this hospital; she should be somewhere else, Angelle smiled at me revealing her dimpled cheeks.

'Dr. Michelle, you are wanted at the forensic ward.'
'I was there two hours ago. Did they tell you why they want me?' I asked, wondering about what could have happened to my patients.

Mostly I dealt with sex offenders, who are rarely seen in good light in society. This is because of the types of crimes they commit; horrid, damning acts which they do on children and those who are vulnerable. Sex offenders are the toughest and perhaps the hardest cases in the criminal justice system, and the harm caused by them make us think of devising further methods for reducing their risk to the community.

From time to time we get appointed from the Courts of Justice to prepare reports, where we assess the individual and aim to offer guidance to justice in its deliberation of the sentence.
The issue is whether these sex offenders are able to continue living in the community without being a risk to themselves and to others. In most cases this is not achieved, as these offenders are brought to court many times. They are very likely to re-offend, even after several years of incarceration; their crimes are serious and at times uncontrollable, so even prison and treatment tend to fail us at times.

SHATTERED WINGS

It is a great burden when it comes to assess these individuals, and for most of the time the weight is on our shoulders. Not only do we assess the individual, but also the risk these individuals pose for the community and their victims. It is not always easy to face this harsh reality. We come face to face with men who senselessly rape women and children, at times without even a slight feeling of remorse inside them.

But, like anything else in life, someone has to deal with these antisocial individuals. Sex Offenders are not all the same, and vary in age, psychological profile, and history of offending. Also, they differ in their level of impulsiveness and persistence. Most sex offenders have their own preferences when it comes to satisfying their impulses, as there are those who desire adults and others who prefer children. In the latter group we find the paedophiles, who direct their sexual impulses to children and even these have their own preferences. With the ever increasing developments on the internet, child pornography is becoming a fast growing business. The use of chatting makes it easier for paedophiles with a range of choices and preferences.

It makes a strange category of clients. So, I found myself confounded in the walls of this mental hospital working in my profession, which is more a vocation. I prepared to leave and told Angelle that I was going to the Forensic Unit. From my office I walked through the long corridors where the walls are cold and gloomy, as if to remind one that this was a hospital, a particular type of hospital tormented by men's perverted thoughts, full of people who are withdrawn from the rest of society because of their perverse thought

Yet, these walls never cease to transport me into the realm of the past, and shivers travel throughout my body as my imagination takes me into other days, into the medieval era. Often, I picture the women incarcerated and treated in the most brutal way, as described by my patients. God almighty! Even the slightest thought shakes my mind like a quivering earthquake.

But why do men keep on abusing women?

Perhaps this could be the one question which kept me in this job. At the age of twenty -five I graduated in medicine and then followed my studies in psychiatry. My career as a psychiatrist saw its beginning around seven years ago, and each new day is no like the other; no two clients are same. Every person has a story to tell.

Now I am thirty- two and my husband, Jason is thirty-five. Jason is a lawyer and we have been married for five years. Most of all, we complimented each other, both of us coming from different disciplines, yet so close.

The pungent smell of antiseptic led me to the ward. The cold walls peered at me as I walked in and a young male nurse approached me.
'What happened, Karl?' I demanded

SHATTERED WINGS

'Dr. Michelle, Alfred has been aggressive again. We gave him sedatives as you ordered.'

'Ok, thanks,' I murmured, and walked with him to the counselling room. Alfred was already there sitting on the armchair, looking deadly pale while staring blankly at the dark sombre walls.

He was in early forties, a large man with short grey hair and pale skin. Somehow, he looked much older than his age, yet his eyes large and brown were bright, rather mischievous. He was engulfed in the fantasies circling in his psyche.

Karl approached him.

'Alfred, Dr. Michelle is here.'

I entered the room and sat down on the chair facing him. He looked at me and then he lowered his head. I made a sign to the nurse and he went out of the room.

Alfred could be very destructive, causing harm to himself and to others, and the slightest stress or agitation could trigger great turmoil inside him, leading to bouts of aggressiveness. Referred to our institution from the criminal court, Alfred was arrested again for interfering with little girls. This time he had raped a young girl. Now the walls of the institution were suffocating him, perhaps making him realise that he had sinned. I hoped.

Unfortunately I did not get what I anticipated, but it was not new to me.

'So, you are back with us, Fred!' I said with a strong tone to my voice.

Alfred looked bitterly at me, and his gaze was chilling, piercing me like blades at the same time melting with desire, for the image conjured in his world was embedded in his cerebral fantasies.

He then spoke slowly.

'I did it again.'

'I know that, and if I am not mistaken you were under supervision. Fred, is this so?

He stopped and looked pensive. Perhaps he was contemplating on the best response to give me. Then he replied.

'Yeah, three bloody years with the doctors stuffing me with pills, and apart from the probation officer, they were very hard on me.'

I looked directly at him.

'So, what do you expect us to do? Applaud you? You have failed, and you failed us.'

Alfred did not answer, but lowered his head as if trying to mask his shame. I wonder if such a thing existed within him.

I tried to control the anger which was steadily building up inside me. Alfred had relapsed again after being given another chance from the court. It was nothing new; this was a vicious cycle which I had to deal with from time to time. We got the same faces, the same names from one year to another. At times I came to the conclusion that these sex offenders really enjoyed what they did, and it was this instigating circumstance which haunted me day and night. What are we doing to stop this violence, to eliminate these acts?

Alfred's lips were forming into words.

'I stopped the medication and then I could not control myself. She was so sweet, smiling at me...'

SHATTERED WINGS

'Who?' I interrupted him, though already guessing to whom he was referring.
'It's that little angel.'

Of course, I had almost forgotten that for him these poor girls were angels. I rose from my seat and moved around the room.
'So, what are you expecting? Alfred, breaking the Supervision Order is serious and you raped the so called precious little angel. Is that right?' My voice was louder reflecting my rage at this man.
He nodded.

From the other side of the room I saw Karl preparing to enter. I made a signal with my head to indicate that I was fine and needed no assistance. Alfred peered at me and his eyes were blazing with fire.
'I could not help it! The little one was looking at me and her round innocent face enticed me.'
Enticing! He said. I tried to figure out how a little child could be enticing to a man of forty years. There was something strange, and not functioning in his mind, what we call as the criminal mind.
'Ok, Fred, so where was the girl?' I asked.
'I will explain. It happened two weeks ago. We were at a party.'
'With whom?' I interrupted.

'I was with Rose, my wife. One of her friends organized a birthday party and I joined her. Well, at some point Rose walked out of the room to get something from the next room and I remained alone in the room. I got bored and decided to smoke a cigarette. Someone entered the room, my wife, I thought, but it wasn't her. A lovely creature swept from heaven walked before my eyes. She had long golden curls and eyes that set my underpants on fire.'

Alfred paused and there was long silence between us. He took a deep breath and sighed whilst his left hand moved downwards towards his pants. I sat down.

'Hey, I know the feeling, now go on please,' I added firmly.

Alfred was watching me intently, his eyes flecked with light of remembrance of that day. I could easily see the pallor of his skin turning into crimson red as he moved his legs a bit and then spoke again. His voice was fading, almost choked.

'Well, I asked her name, and she told me that her name was Clothilde. 'Nice name,' I uttered whilst I moved from my seat, got rid of the cigarette and I walked closer. This blue eyed baby appeared to me like the sea, promising desire. I could see the hidden lust within her combined with innocence. Oh, my body ached as I played with her hair. 'You hair is beautiful.' I sighed as I longed to smell its freshness. 'My mother did it for me,' she answered. 'And where is your mother now?' She pouted her lips. 'She is with papa in the other room.' 'Ok', I said. That meant I had to be fast, this little nymphet was taunting me, her soft pale skin was urging me on under her light linen dress.

SHATTERED WINGS

I continued listening to Alfred s' version now feeling calmer.

Alfred sighed and then continued, and then the sparkle in his eyes said it all.

'Doctor Michelle, I made her sit down and she moved her legs. My God! What pain, an exhilarating pain between my thighs. My pants became tight as I felt a shiver running all over my spine and a feeling of fire heating up in my head. You know the feeling well, it's when you feel the heat for your man.'

'Alfred, we are here to talk about you,' I said firmly.

'Sorry, doctor, but even thinking of it sends shivers all over my whole being and yes I will go on. My body was smarting with pain, an inner passion which longed to emerge. Her thighs were soft as silk. I asked her, 'Clothilde, do you want to play with me?' She nodded which I took for a yes. For me it meant her approval for touching her inner velvet. She wanted to play, and play I would. My body was still aching for her. I plucked up my courage and did it to my little Clothilde. My head was racing with drums humming all over my head.

The tighter she was the more she increased my pulsating desire. I covered her mouth with my hands whilst thrusting myself between her soft thighs. She could not take it, she was small and my thing was hurting her. The soft flower inside of her was opening up and tearing her into pieces. It was hurting her, she started screaming, but her mouth was securely covered. It was hurting me more with the deep pleasure running all over me. I was all over the moon. And that was it. A knock on the door and my heart pounded, I wanted to move but the pleasure was amusingly strong and left me motionless. Then they caught me, and my passion play stopped abruptly here.'

Poor little angel! What she had to go through because of this monster of a man. A cold shiver ran all over my scalp as I thought of the girl. Suddenly, I recalled the reports and scenes I witnessed when I was a junior doctor. Sexual abused children were admitted to the Emergency Department for examination and it was incredibly hard not to reveal any emotion. These children had severe injuries and the psychological trauma would remain with them for years if not for a lifetime. Now, Clothilde had had the same fate and I was here with the author of her sufferings. Alfred. I turned my focus to him.

'And you are back with us, under arrest,' I affirmed.

'Yeah,' he responded.

'Exactly, what is best for you, and you stand little chance.'

'But you will help me, won't you?'

'You d have to help yourself first.'

'I am a ruined man.'

'You need therapy.'

'Will therapy ever control my passions?'

'You have no other alternative, Fred.'

Alfred lowered his head thoughtfully. He had no other way but to succumb. He looked straight at me.

'Doctor Michelle, will you help me at court?'

'I will state only the facts, nothing else.'

'I will do as you tell me.'

SHATTERED WINGS

Could he be trusted? Well, Alfred was trying to give me what I wanted to hear.

Yet, I was prompted to ask him, 'Alfred, why do you keep on doing this? You know you are hurting innocent people.'

He lowered his head and pondered on these words. 'I know, but can't help it. It is something which is beyond me.'

'But tell me, don't you feel remorse for hurting the girl.'

He stared at me and then uttered.

'I wish I could stop, but when the urge comes I feel helpless and lost, as if a monster has taken over me. All I can feel is the pain which does not leave me till I do it...'

'Ok, Alfred,' I said, interrupting him. I prepared to go.

That was all, he felt overpowered by this tormenting desire which drove him. I left him in the cold room wrapped in his warm fantasies, a voyage which he willingly succumbed to. He had no choice but to revert to the world he knew so well, a world which awakened his heart but generated destructive seeds of pain in other's hearts.

How could one concur with this reality? These were men who directed their sexual urges towards children and vulnerable people. Was it illness which impelled them to act in this appalling way towards children or was it driven by malicious intent?

It is very difficult to diagnose what sex offending really is. The child molesters and paedophiles are one of these types, as seen in Alfred's case. He felt defenceless with children, more vulnerable than the victim. Alfred s' sexual urges for children know their origin from his childhood days and I knew that deep inside him there was motivation to change his path of desires. Yet, he never succeeded.

This was the fourth case of sexual assault on children, the first case being that of raping his three- year old daughter and who is now in care order. Rose, his wife, left him and asked for a separation, but then went back to him, said she felt sorry for him and that after all he was the man of her life.

This was a concept which I could never comprehend or agree with. Alfred derived his sexual satisfaction from forcing himself inside little girls, and yet, at the same time, he continued having sexual relations with his wife, but he confessed that the former gave him more pleasure.

Nevertheless, these perverted sexual urges had their origin in his childhood. It is a rather sad story which had its strong implications throughout his life. Alfred was a young school boy of eight years when he was sexually assaulted by one of his teachers, and that opened the pathway to where he is now. He was in a tender age where he could be easily influenced and would already have started to explore his genitals, which is part of the development process. This process was interrupted

SHATTERED WINGS

by another monster, who initiated Alfred to this vicious circle. Sexual assault is a common serious harm that achild can experience. Sex offenders come into many categories such as exhibitionists, paedophile, the rapist, sexual sadist, sexual murderer, violent predator. Through their behaviour we determine the level of dangerousness.

Certain categories must be viewed with caution as many sex offenders have multiple paraphilias.
Amongst them I would mention, the rape forced sexual contact, child molesting having sexual contact with a person under eighteen years of age.
Also, the exposing and displaying of one s' genitals for the purpose of sexual gratification and voyeurism which is watching someone for the purpose of sexual gratification amongst many.

Mr.X was a teacher in his early fifties who showed great interest and dedication to his students, but that was only a mask to cover his other perverted inclinations. Often, he took his students on cultural tours and organized outings for with the idea of breaking away from their studies. A noble idea, but his intentions were far from that, and originated from his deviant sexual urges. Yet, no one had any idea what was he up to. On one of these outings, Alfred and his sister joined the group and they all had a good time in each other s' company. Then it was time to go back. Mr. X approached Alfred and patted him on his shoulder.
'Alfred, I would like to show you a new game of soldiers, the ones you like.'
'Yes, sir,' Alfred said meekly.

'Would you come to my office?'

'But mama will be waiting.'

'Tell your sister to tell her you are going to be in my company.'

'Ok,'

So, Alfred joined his teacher, hoping to see a new game and indeed there was a new game waiting for him. The teacher took him to his house and led him to the office. The house was deserted at that time and all was still but for the slow movements of the clock. Mr. X moved closer to Alfred.

'We will soon start,' he uttered, 'Now, I want you to do as I say. If you obey me you will get a lot of privileges.'

He then stroked Alfred's cheeks and said, 'You are a special boy. I presume your mother and father tell you this.'

'No, never, sir,' Alfred answered innocently.

'But you are special.'

Then he asked Alfred to sit down on the chair and then brought a rope a bound Alfred's hands. Alfred looked at him with fear in his eyes, but then Mr. X caressed his face, which soothed him a bit. This was not to Alfred's advantage, but rather to his teacher.

'Do not be afraid, it will be ok. I have chosen you for this game, but this is between you and me. Ok?'

Then he asked Alfred to open his legs while sitting.

'Imagine being the best in class, your mother will be very proud of you. Don't you think?'

Alfred nodded.

Mr. X stroked his hair.

'Good boy.'

'But can I see the game?' Alfred insisted.

'It is coming.'
Alfred nodded again and the most bizarre game commenced.
Mr. X moved closer to Alfred and asked him to spread his legs a bit, unzipped his pants and then played with his genitals. Alfred tried to speak, but Mr. X covered his mouth.
'You like it, Alfred. Tell me you like it.'
Alfred was petrified and had no other alternative but to accept and subdue to his teacher. After all, Mr. X was a good teacher and was rather pleased with the favours and special attention he thought he was receiving. Mr. X was his role model and ultimately Alfred believed that this was all right. Disgusting and shameful abuse!

These encounters were more frequent, and every time Alfred was being introduced to new games followed by more games. Also, Alfred was then introduced to Child Pornography. These hideous experiences were kept in the dark. So, the abuse went on in utter silence and no one wondered what was going on. One, evening Alfred had to be taken to hospital complaining of digestive problems. While examining the boy, the doctor noticed that the enlarged cavity of his anus. This was the result of the countless times of Alfred being sodomised by this monster. There are signs and symptoms to indicate that children are being abused. Some children start withdrawing from the rest of the family, often run away. Also, they have nightmares and wet their beds. If they are being penetrated vaginally or anal they will find it difficult to walk or sit down. They will complain of pain and have problems with urinating or even can contract venereal diseases. There were cases where children acted in a seductive way in the presence of other adults, or demonstrate unusual sexual knowledge.

In the case of Alfred the medical examination threw light on the facts and the secret was unmasked. Alfred was unknowingly yielding to this abuse, in the hope of getting special attention in return. Mr. X was then caught and no one could postulate these incidents, due to the fact that Mr. X was considered a respectable man and one of the best teachers. Yet the damage inflicted on Alfred was irreversible and the monster created another one. Many years later, exactly when Alfred was fifteen years old, he raped a girl of eight years, but somehow he got away with it. Some years later he met Rose, who is now his wife. He married her, hoping to solve this problem. This was not destined to work, and Alfred ended up raping his three year old daughter. This was a tragic episode, but perhaps this was the only fact which instilled the feeling of remorse within him and in one of my sessions he once cried, touched by a wave of despair.

'I just cannot help it,' he accounted, 'Every time I see a little angel I get those chills inside of me, urging me to go inside her. Her pain alleviates the pain I feel inside me. It's burning tearing me apart.'

There is no explanation; children remind Alfred of his past when he himself was assaulted in the most bizarre way. The experience of pain is instilled within him. I walked away pondering on what he had just told me, trying to conceive this mystery. What I mused about was the fact that there wasn't any solution at hand.

These offenders needed to be controlled in the community, or in institutions, and the only hope which resided inside me was the concept of treatment and psychotherapy. Through therapy we aim to find the clues which divert their sexual passion towards children.

These retrospective thoughts lingered with me throughout the few moments after my session with Alfred as I walked away from the ward. My encounter with these patients taught me that most paedophiles have more than one victim, almost having sex with more children and for them it is a gratification boosting their hungry ego. These incorrigible human creatures say they prefer young children to avoid the risk of pregnancy and infections. It is not a novelty to find amongst them teachers, church members, coaches, care workers, photographers, most likely in circumstances involving children. Also, most often the offender was known to the family or related directly to the victim.

Church members involved in paedophilia are not uncommon, but the latter meddle with children in the absence of females. Still it is not right. Well, that is what I hope. The question which we often ask ourselves is whether these child molesters were abused when they were children. In fact, there are a percentage of children who were abused in their childhood and then ended up molesting other children when they became adults. This abuse provokes another cycle, where the victim becomes the abuser as a way to relieve the inner tension or to appease the inner conflict and repressed emotions kindled by sexual abuse.

On the other side of the coin there were also children who were sexually abused and grew up as normal adults.
Another fraction which we cannot omit is the female offenders. These cases might be under-reported, but there were incidences of abuses, though we tend to disbelieve that these types of offenders do really exist.

Yet, studies indicate that there are also a small percentage of women offenders. In certain cases women were accomplices in bringing victims forward to the aggressors. Even men get sexually abused by other men, and even by women, but are less willing to report this crime. For some young men, being sexually abused by an older woman is instead seen as a compliment.

Rapists form another group of sex offenders, although paedophiles do rape children. Rape is a word which in itself inflicts agonizing pain which we choose to create myths around the topic. This horrendous crime affects everyone under the sun, but unfortunately it is directed to us women and children. It has been with us and it will remain so.

SHATTERED WINGS

The thought of it sends tremors all over my body and an extract from a book, which I read during my studies, had a great impact on me. It fascinated me and terrified me at the same time, as it dealt with the ruthless treatment of women in medieval times. It's a devastating reality which afflicted those poor women, who were raped, abused and then burned at the stake. A fraction of women in our times are still vulnerable and subject to men's power. This notion will continue to haunt me, residing in my memories, but I believe that every woman should keep it in her mind. This deadly, devastating crime can come like a thief in the night. Above all, rape is the violation of the most private parts of a woman's body, and even her self. It is an act of power over women, but an act which inflicts deep trauma on the victim. At times, this devastating crime puts the victim under trial instead of the rapists. Yet rape has been with us from the beginning of humanity, wherever men used their virility as a means of exerting power over women. Rape in times of war is another common crime. It is a common phenomenon, showing lack of discipline, and is in most cases used as a tactic of terror and revenge. Many girls and women have been singled out for rape and torture.

These atrocities leave me dumbfounded, especially when these incidents are documented in recent history. A cold shudder ran all over me as I thought of the numerous cases of rapes during wars. And I think of the horrifying rapes by Nazi officials, where women were often raped while being kept prisoners in the concentration camps. Then there were the

Russians after the downfall of Berlin at the end of World War II, and more recently in Bosnia and also in Iraq.

On one of my trips to Germany, to Berlin, I could not but think of its historical events. This interesting and beautiful city is enriched with culture and important remnants of history which influenced the world. But, it was a daunting memory which oppressed me, for behind the cultural buildings I was recalling the appalling cries of thousands of women. After the war, the city of Berlin had to witness more pain inflicted on her people. The year of 1945 was supposed to bring utter relief from the cruelty inflicted by the Nazi's, but instead it witnessed another horrible nightmare. At the time the Soviets arrived in Berlin, it was the women who suffered most, and few women in Berlin managed to escape the lust of the Red Army as the Soviet troops were called. Thousands of Berliners were raped over and over again, with numerous stories by those who managed to survive, but there were those who committed suicide.

For those wretched soldiers, these sexual assaults are just a little fun which they deserve. The mention of the Red Army sends chills up and down the spines of old Berliner women who were present at that period. That was one part of my recollections of Berlin, but surely there were other beautiful memories of the city which I cherish. But without knowing the shadow of my patients cannot leave my path.

SHATTERED WINGS

The reality of sexual offences still haunts us and whatever we say or do, rape keeps occurring. Still, we seek to comprehend what goes through the mind of men, the channel from their minds to their impulses urging them to react in such a way. Whatever, they are with us, confronting us with their acts.

Rapists are another category of sex offenders who are hard to work with, like any other sex offenders they boast by using brute force to enforce their control on those who subject to their aggression. These types of offenders never assume responsibility for their actions, and deny any involvement. They want us to believe that they were right and that all men would behave in the same way if confronted with the same situation. It is always the victim who provoked them and they present numerous excuses to justify their actions. They would tell you bluntly; she was too sexy, too vulnerable or, she walked, looked and dressed in such a way. In other words they were provoked by her or by him. Anyone can be raped, from nuns to whores; but certainly rapists do have their choices where they look for all type of vulnerability.

In most cases, rapes were pre- planned. Offenders have spent time fantasising and premeditating the action. In other instances it just happened. When it comes to treatment, there are many alternatives, and they include psycho-surgery, castration, drug therapy and counselling therapies.

Our aim is to help them control their behaviour by being honest with themselves and take responsibility for their actions and also understanding the effects on their victims. My patients need to learn how to handle their anger and solve their problems without reverting to force. That would enable them to re integrate in the community.

Rapists are classified in various categories. For instance, we get the power assertive rapist who rapes as to declare his masculine power, to dominate and impose his virility over women. He believes he must get it.
These types of offenders claim that they have weapons, but they only do this to ensure that the victim is petrified. Thus, the victim cooperates with him out of fear and terror. These types are the most common.

Then we get the power reassurance rapist, who rapes women to compensate for his sexual inadequacy. He strives to control women and puts them in situations where they cannot repel him. The anger retaliation rapist rapes out of revenge and hatred for women. He aims to humiliate their victims and discredit them. He has got to punish women, and in such cases this type of rapist might injure his victims to the point of needing medical intervention. Another type of rapist is the anger excitation rapist who is thrilled by the suffering he inflicts on his victim. This is the sadistic type who excites himself by creating pain and torture in his victim. This type is the most dangerous and often the victim is killed.

Then there are the opportunity rapists and these are the ones who take the opportunity to rape, often this is done in conjunction with other crime such as robbery, burglary or kidnapping. Rape in juveniles is not uncommon. These young offenders have problems with authority, the police and justice and seek to project their anger by punishing victims and proving their masculinity. Why all this? It is a dilemma which will haunt us constantly and will remain us for more years.

I returned to my office. The rain has increased now, beating on my window as if in complete harmony with the drumming in my silent thinking. Then, I take at Alfred's file, which was in the cabinet and write the usual report, describing briefly the last session I have had with him. Alfred had to be imprisoned and administered with life long treatment. At least it will ensure protection for him and his victims.

His victims…would they ever find peace? I thought of the little angel, as he called her. Certainly, her days are different now, tormented by the nightmare Alfred devised for her, and she will recall scene by scene and every minute is a journey heading towards a bottomless pit.

Whereas for my patient, those moments were a glimpse of paradise, for his little angel one single thought of the event will plunge her into the deepest

hell. Yes, these victims' reality fell like scattering drops of rain deep inside me, deeper than the rain beating heavily on the window.
The effects are endless almost for a lifetime.

A case which comes in mind is that of Jimmy, he could be referred as the anger retaliation rapist.
His contemplated gaze prevailed contempt, which he suppressed inside him for years. Whenever I look at him I see his eyes blazing with fire, exasperated for what he had to go through because of his mother. He hated all women, above all his mother, whom he blamed for all his distress. Jimmy was thirty nine, large with curly hair and penetrating dark eyes. He was serving a prison sentence for rape.

I recall the sheer coldness of his tone whilst he spoke in one of my sessions.
'It's her fault; the bitch,' he stated with anger in his voice. His eyes were like daggers piercing ruthlessly, as if instead of me there was his mother sitting before him and not the therapist. No, doubt she would get her just desert from him. But she was not there, and I was sitting in her stead. I sat there motionless, trying to control myself as he was about to start his story.

Jimmy s' mother was a prostitute and as soon as he was born she sent him to a children's home. When Jimmy was five years old, his mother took him again with her, exposing him to the kind of life she lived. Every night she was visited by various men and whilst Jim was supposed to be asleep he was allured to sexual practices.

'One night, I could not sleep, but kept hearing voices as if someone was in my room. I tried to close my eyes and sleep again. Suddenly, a pair of hands grabbed me and covered my mouth. He was a man, one of those who visited my mother. He came into my room.'

Jimmy panted, breathless. Silence reigned between us. Then Jimmy continued.

'This strange man was watching me, scrutinizing me for quite a while. Then his gaze moved to my lower body. He moved closer and touched the part between my thighs and then he showed me something. 'Look at this, Jimmy. How about having some play?' It was repulsive and I looked away but he persisted. 'This will give you energy boy. It will make you a man.' He then touched my thighs and then I felt a surging pleasure between my thighs. Yet, he moved further and made me turn my back. I felt a burning sensation, a shiver running all over my spine. He pulled down my pants and was pressing me closer and closer. Again, he pressed the thing in my behind, in my anus. There was more pain and pain like daggers inside me.'

Jimmy lowered his head, clutching his fists.

'So, this went on,' I remarked.

'Yes, he kept coming every night, messing with me. I could not tell my mother. The man said he would kill me if I dared open my mouth. Every night he had sex with my mother and than came to play with me.'

So that was it. Jimmy was initiated into sexual abuse. He grew up with mixed emotions, detesting all women, desiring them at the same time. Women have become a source of hatred and revenge against his mother. Jimmy blamed his mother. According to Jimmy, his mother knew what was happening to him, and still she kept it hidden, letting him suffer. All women had to suffer, and this was expressed in the brutal way he raped women. This was rather a distorted philosophy which was revealed by him.

At the age of eighteen Jimmy had a relationship with a pretty young woman. All was well till one day he violently raped her after an argument he had with her. Jimmy was then sentenced to six years in prison. Once, out of prison, Jimmy resorted to crime again, and violent rape has become a habit. One evening he broke into a house where a young girl was alone after her parents
had gone out. Someone knocked on the door, and thinking that her parents returned, she went to open the door.

She found Jimmy and he told her not to be afraid and that he did not want to harm her nor rob her. She struggled to send him away but he was already in. Then Jimmy pushed her back and forced sex on her, forcing her to do it in as many different positions as he pleased. The girl was only eleven, and Jimmy forced himself in her genitals and anus till the girl bled.

SHATTERED WINGS

That same night Jimmy had introduced this young girl to the nightmare which he experienced in earlier in his life. He was sentenced again to prison, but released five years later for good behaviour. Again, Jimmy was out in the community, no supervision, no treatment. He was in his early thirties when he raped a six year old girl, an endless episode of sadistic pain. The girl was torn, with grave injuries in her genital area.

I still recall the feeling of revulsion when I went through his court report. This man has turned into a monster who indulged in creating nightmares for others. In one of my sessions I asked Jimmy if he had any remorse or any feeling for what he did.
'No. '
'Why?' I asked, though not surprised.
Jimmy gazed at me, unmoved but the anger in his eyes was inscrutable.
'No, she just got what she asked for, as her body was aching to be touched and fondled. These little buds like to be fondled and touched by me.'
'You have harmed the girl,' I said hoping to get a different response.
'No, the pain passes quickly, a little pain and then pleasure, a burning sensation swarming all over my veins. It's a flood of sweet feelings.'
'That s' what you were taught as a child.'
Silence! It was only silence which dominated the cold, old room, but I was certain that deep inside him there was an agonizing pain and a torturous interplay of emotions. His past was pulsating in his veins, and with my words I had taken him on a voyage inside his soul, through his experience of

sexual abuse. This abuse has blocked his sensitivity, and now he had become like a walking machine, controlled by his phallus.

He hoped to get a better chance from court. He did not get it, and I was relieved as it was what we were hoping from court. These men created victims each hour of the day, the reverse of art.
Yet, I marvel at the imminent contrast between those devoted artists who gave up their possessions and almost their life, to give us a new birth of beauty, and my patients who only create devastating pain and misery. Submerged in this reality I kept working in my office.

The next day the sun returned back to our offices and with the glaring rays the view from my window the hospital appeared different, less sombre. It might not change the gloom and the inner painful torments experienced by my patients, but at least the sun helped to alleviate this feeling.
I sipped the rest of the coffee on my desk and prepared to go out to court. Today, I had to present Alfred's report.

The court of Justice lay in the central region of the capital city, Valletta. It is a huge building with enormous columns reminding one of its grandiosity. The corridors were overcrowded where all sorts of people gathered; the defendants and their families, victims, police officers, experts, witnesses, and others were all waiting impatiently for their turn. Some looked grievously serious, others with no expression at all. I stood there watching people pondering over the case. Then I was called in to testify. I could see Alfred sitting in the first row of the benches, allocated for the accused.

The magistrate asked that all those present leave the room while I went to take the oath prior to submitting my report. The Magistrate addressed me and asked to state verbally what my conclusions were. I stated that my patient had a problem in controlling his sexual impulses, and that he needed psychiatric treatment and psychotherapy. His defence counsel wanted my opinion whether or not he should be given another opportunity in the community. I frowned and tried to mask my disapproval. That would be the gravest mistake, as this was not the case with my patient, not in this situation. I firmly stated that my patient was a great risk to society and was not yet prepared for life in the community. Wisely, the prosecution officer reminded the court that my patient broke the conditions of a Supervision Order given by on previous occasions.

The Magistrate ordered a Treatment Order, and Alfred was to be institutionalised until we decide his readiness for going back in the community. The victims also have a hard time in court. Women and children have to retell their experiences by detail, which is traumatic, invoking many painful emotions and memories which will remain throughout their lives. Alfred, a victim who turned into a perpetrator, was now in our hands.

There is a question which is very hard to answer and that is how we identify a rapist, stalker or an abuser? It is impossible to predict who will be a potential rapist, but there may be traits which might be important to look at for, as they might be a predominant indication of sexual assault. One should be aware if a man suddenly starts acting strange or showing certain traits, for instance, insensitivity to others. In this case the person puts a lot of emphasis on himself, and his needs become extremely important. Such a person has no understanding and thinks that the world owes him and makes his partner feels bad for not doing what he wants. Also, if the person makes nasty or degrading comments about others, looks down on others and feels superior.

Another type of person may use hostile and threatening language and these may be the men who refer to women as bitches. They have no respect for females. Someone who uses bullying as threats to get his way, will most likely resort to violence to get what he wants and sexual violence is one of aspect of this. Excessive anger and the way a person reacts to anger is another factor. For instance, a person may explode abruptly and manifest his anger in abuse and even rape.
Other factors are alcohol and drug abuse, as an intoxicated person has no inhibitors as regards violence and sex. An obsessive person is another signal to be aware of. This is a man who will not leave women alone and can force her to be intimate, and his anger may escalate if his

advances are rejected. Some of my cases showed these traits.

Rape and sexual abuse in mental institutions is not uncommon, where mental patients are raped by staff or in such rare cases by other male patients. Mental patients are most vulnerable and less likely to be believed due to their diagnostic illnesses. For instance, patients suffering from Schizophrenia or with delusional illness are rarely believed when they report an incidence of sexual abuse. Most often, the event is regarded as part of the delusion, adding to more frustration to these patients.

A case which I recall is that of a woman in her early thirties: Caroline. She suffered from severe depression and had a drinking problem. Caroline s' marriage was not functioning and whenever she drank, which was on daily basis, she became aggressive. This went on and on until it became so bad, for her own protection, Caroline was admitted in a mental hospital. Whilst hospitalized, Caroline seemed to be improving. She responded well to treatment and attended to Psychotherapy.

All was going well, but then this improvement was suddenly interrupted by an unexpected sudden event and Caroline reverted back to her situation. It happened one afternoon by the person she least expected. Caroline was walking back to her ward after a session at the Occupational Therapy room, which was quite near the Female ward. Caroline was on her way when she head someone calling her name. She looked back and saw Benjamin, a nurse attendant. Benjamin was in his late thirties, quite a nice man, large and was friendly with everyone including the patients. It was good to see a smiling face in a place like this. Yet, Benjamin's motives were far from that. That day he greeted Caroline as usual.

'Hi, Caroline,' he started by saying.
'Hello,' she replied, 'I am going to the ward.'
'Do you want me to show you the new puppy?' Benjamin insisted.
Caroline accepted and followed him, eager to see this new puppy. Such circumstances outside the ward were rare. Instead of leading her to the puppy, Benjamin took Caroline in a small room at the end of the deserted corridor. Benjamin stroked her cheeks.
'Caroline, I find you very attractive,' he said.
But Caroline wanted to see the puppy, he promised her.
'I want to see the puppy,' she told him.
'Soon, my dear,'
'Where is it?'
Then Benjamin asked her to close her eyes while he brings the puppy. Unaware what was next, Caroline obeyed him and closed her eyes and the next thing she knew Benjamin's large body was close to hers. Panic seized her and Caroline made an attempt to release herself, but did not succeed. Benjamin covered her mouth whilst swiftly touching her breasts and thighs. Then he tore her underwear and forced himself fiercely inside her. When he was finished with her, Benjamin arranged her

clothes and then said to her mockingly, 'A word about this and you'll be screwed.'

Caroline was shocked, but still found the courage to slap him on his cheeks.

'No one will believe you, anyway.'

Then Benjamin walked away leaving Caroline panic stricken, disbelieving what had happened to her. With great effort Caroline returned to the ward and immediately informed the Staff about this incident, but Caroline was hardly believed. Benjamin was very well respected and no one suspected that he could go that far. When confronted by the Hospital's Administration, Benjamin denied any involvement and told them that Caroline encouraged his advances. Benjamin was not charged whilst Caroline was transferred in a more controlled ward.

Benjamin went on with his job until he did it again, and this time luck was not on his side to conceal his deceit. His impulses went far beyond him and this time Benjamin attempted rape on an Occupational Therapist. That was it. Soon after this incident, Caroline's case was revised and during Interrogation, Benjamin admitted to having raped Caroline.

It is such an unfortunate fate for patients and other people in vulnerable situations. Yet, there are other situations which are almost hard to register. At that moment I thought of another vulnerable situation, and that was Anita's case. Anita's case differed from that of Caroline. Anita was sixteen years old and came from an upper social class, with her father occupying a very high position in the Administration of an important Department. She had everything a girl of her age could ask for. Her father was very well respected but behind the good image he portrayed there was an obscure reality overshadowing Anita s' life.

The real truth was devastatingly shocking. For ten whole years, he was abusing his two children Anita and Michael, two years older than Anita. All this happened in silence and none of the children dared speak up about this situation. But, when Michael turned eighteen, he decided to leave home and go and work abroad. Michael asked his sister to join him, but Anita refused out of fear and because of her studies. The sexual abuse went on in deep silence and her father used to lock her in her bedroom, controlling her life. Yet, this saga had to come to an end and one day, whilst at school, Anita opened up with one of the teachers who reported the case.

Being aware of this, Anita's father took immediate action against his daughter in an attempt to stop her from tarnishing his reputation. To punish her, he signed for his daughter to be admitted into a mental hospital, where she was certified as suffering from Multiple Personality.

Anita kept on repeating the same version of the story and the case was followed. Her brother Michael was called back to give his version of the story, which eventually led to their father being accused for sexually abusing his son and daughter.

Sad but real! It is amazing how far people can go and how many innocent people end up being victims of this cruelty, most often in long deep silence.

These were my thoughts on my way from Court and when I got back there was another interesting case demanding my attention. This was different. On the desk there was a note on the desk from Angelle. *Dr. Albert would like to speak to you.*

Dr. Albert was the Head of Psychiatry. I wrote some notes in Alfred's file and prepared to leave.
The head office is situated in the central building. I knocked on the door and entered in the room. Dr. Albert was in his late forties, and had been the head of Psychiatry for almost fifteen years. He was the one who distributed cases to us. Since he called me in his office I figured out that there was another case and most likely another report from court. I was right.
'Sit down. Dr. Michelle,' he started by saying.
I sat down.
'Dr. Michelle, I am assigning you another case.'
'Yes?' I replied. Of course, I knew, whilst thinking of the piles of files on my desk.
Dr. Albert looked at me behind his spectacles. He was watching me intently and then he spoke again.
'This time it is a woman.'
I took a deep breath. A woman!

This sounded interesting; we rarely get women offenders.

'Is it the same offence?'

'No, not exactly as you are thinking. This case differs from others, by the simple fact that the young woman is a victim of rape.'

'A victim of rape?' I asked him rather surprised. 'We rarely get reports on rape.'

'Precisely! In this case the victim committed a crime. She murdered her perpetrator.'

I sat back amazed, but I tried to remain calm and detached. It must have been very tough for her to end up this way.

'Poor girl,' I exclaimed, 'where is she, now?'

'She is in prison. Her jury will commence within a month, and the presiding judge wants us to prepare a report.'

There were many questions, as we rarely got these types of report before a jury.

'Forgive me, Dr. Albert, but I I have never given a report before the jury.' I told him.

'I know, but this is a special case.'

'Ok then. I will start straight away.' I replied.

He nodded and seemed satisfied with my response. I then thanked him and walked out of the room. My mind was overwhelmed by a deluge of thoughts, and a sense of pity for this woman took over me. I tried to imagine what she had to go through whilst I recalled every scene, detail by detail as described by my patients. Now, the victims were closer than I thought. Confronting me was the truth of rape and it was going to be tough, I said to myself.

Looking from my window, what I saw was not the rain, nor the glittering rays of sunlight, but the harshness of rape.

That same afternoon I went to prison, to the female wing where I was going to start working with the victim and enter her world, which revealed more to me than I was expecting. This was an astounding recount of pain, suffering and degradation which a woman can go through. It is the reality which, at times, we would rather bury and omit from our everyday lives. I faced this reality day by day, one after the other.

She entered in the room accompanied by two prison officers. From the way she walked I could see she was reluctant. Francine, walked with her head lowered down, and then she looked at me. She had the most beautiful eyes. I have ever seen, big velvety brown eyes, beaming but mournful.
'Good day Francine. I am Dr. Michelle.'
She stared at me, scrutinizing me.
'Are you from court?' she asked. Her voice was low and soft.
'I will be preparing a report for court.'
My words seemed to console her a bit. She sat down and looked at me.
'For what?' she asked innocently.
'Francine, what you will be telling me will be presented to the court, but only to help you.' she nodded and that meant that I could go on.

'Ok.'
'What you will be telling me will remain confidential and will only be presented with your permission.'
She took a deep breath. She looked helpless as if she could not belong here. I wanted to help her. Her eyes were hiding the pain and sorrow inflicted by the act.

Francine s' story starts from here. It was a different version from the ones I get from my patients. It is a real account woven from the threads of agony. A memory with a wound which only time can heal.

The woman before me was the mirror of this Hell.

SHATTERED WINGS

FRANCINE

There are days which are full of light and this light remains with us for days. Other days are dark and gloomy, as if weaved in the womb of Hell. These days are the ones which linger in my unconscious, taunting me like an augur of the tormenting soul I longed to forget; and here I am in this world of despair and darkness. Loneliness took the plunge over me and I found myself drowned into a sea of utter loneliness and pain, as my memories take me to that murky evening.

Strange, how fate can be our mistress and take us through passages of events which determine our direction of events. Moment by moment our life is being constructed and sculpted on clay and its memories engraved in our soul are rewriting our story, my story. I often marvel at mine. There is no end or beginning. From where shall I start?

It is a long story which does not pertain my past, but still it is a part of myself and my past.
I look at the warm gaze of Dr Michelle and though I refused her coming here, now that I have looked into her eyes I feel different. Here, in prison, one learns not to trust at times not even ones own self and your next step. They betray you. Yet, this woman's eyes were warm, they melted the wall in my heart hardened by experiences.

I plucked up my courage and started to speak. There are two persons inside me, the innocent girl and the woman who is the murderer, but I will commence with the story of the girl. I was twenty two years old when I was raped and since then my life took another turn and changed completely.

The sky now is blurred with heavy clouds which overshadow my thoughts. I am another woman now. Before the rape life was a flowing river full of promises and dreams. All was within my reach written on silver clouds. Everything was within my reach, written on silver clouds. I had everything I could ask for and the best way to start my story is from the period after my studies. I lived with my family in a village in the central part of Malta. My father was an engineer and my mother a nurse. That was till she married. I had an older brother who was studying for an engineer following my father. I took after my mother.

My father was also a great lover of history and he made sure that we got as much information as we could about the history of Malta. Well, the island is embodied with the remnants of different cultures, which fascinated me from my early introduction to the history. From my early years I grew to love it. My first encounter was with the Neolithic Temples and this was done through regular visits to the place. There was an era of mystery which surmounted these stones and from the very first day I wanted to know more about them, who built them, why and how. I only got a few answers, but surely I was fortunate to be blessed with a father like mine, for this gave me an advantage at school and I knew more than the rest of the girls in class. There was a time in my school days when I thought of studying history, to learn and perhaps discover what was really behind those majestic temples who have become my friends.

But my career had to be nursing.

My first nursing placement, after successfully completing my studies, was in a medical ward. Medical wards were rather hectic, but interesting where we got many cases of heart diseases, lung cancer, leukaemia, chest infections and other serious illnesses. This was rather generic, but this gave me enough time to acquire experience and then decide in which area to specialize if I were ever to continue nursing.

We considered every patient as an individual who needed our full attention, and we had patients of all ages. Coming face to face with the younger patients really grieved me. To come across young patients with serious illnesses, sometimes leading to death, when they didn't know was difficult. This burden was hard to carry at times. We read reports, read the diagnosis and were trained in matters which enabled us to foresee the end results, as well as working close with doctors.

There were days overcrowded by gloom which descended upon me like black clouds and I had to stop and ponder.

Why all the suffering and pain?

Physical pain could be devastating and this was reflected in the vague gaze of the patients. Whilst medicating them or helping them I could not look directly into their eyes without sensing this pain as well as their never ending questions, most often with no answer. I endeavoured to smile when in my heart I felt like crying. Yet, we were thought to keep hoping, till the last moment, till the last breath.

The team of doctors in our ward did their best to prolong the lives of our patients fighting against hope, most of the time losing the battle. Professor Henry Borg was one of the Consultants, a large man well in his fifties, firm but kind. He demanded respect, but respected us too and had time to listen to us. Professor Borg's courage and diligence inspired me and we used to spend hours discussing concepts and theories and he was always open to new ideas and suggestions and always ready for new insights. From his part he encouraged me to continue on with my studies and to specialize in the area of nursing.

Still I was not sure for one of my aspirations was to become a doctor. It was still a possibility. Yet, fate had a different path for me and an event could blur one's route. It was not only my road which was halted, but there were other individuals whom I encountered everyday.

We somehow think that we can modify our fate and that of those we love, like we do with our patients. Every day we hoped to take hold of our patients' fate and mould it for their best, but contrary to our expectations, there were other forces working against us.

It is a shattering cold reality and too hard to register, maybe never ever to accept the budding life being destructed, overtaken by the angel of death. I wonder for how many times I crossed his path. He walked each night in our ward whispering in someone's ear, and then the next day he or she will be his victim.

There were times when it was unbearably hard to accept this unfolding reality. Like the case of Stephanie. This case taught me about the harshness of death and no matter how I endeavoured to escape from his claws, he was there staring at us. Stephanie was sixteen years old, beautiful and always smiling, and was admitted into our ward suffering from chest pain. Stephanie was still young and had no history of cardiovascular problems, not even in her family.

Professor Borg wanted to do more investigations, so she remained for more time in our ward. That gave me more time to be with her as she often called me to go and sit beside her.

'Come Miss Francine,' she said one afternoon smiling as she always did. I admired her. She never complained and was always smiling; her eyes were always shining with hope. For me, that was enough, instilling a ray of hope in their smile was the ultimate mission. I sat beside her and she smiled and then her beautiful mouth formed into words.

'When will this pass?'

'Soon,' I uttered while holding her hand firmly.

A shiver ran all over my spine and a strange feeling overpowered me.

I only learned later.

Then she discussed her plans for the future. Stephanie wanted to study Psychology.

'Miss Francine, one day I'll be a Psychologist working in a mental hospital.'

'Of course you will,' I added, whilst thinking of those poor souls in hospital These people were vulnerable and needed help, but now God was sending an angel to help them. Will she make it? For, I much feared that another angel would come and take her before time. I hoped that I had been wrong. But I admired this sweet lovely patient who was bequeathed with noble thoughts for others even though she was afflicted by pain and disease.

She smiled, her eyes full of hope hiding the inner twinge of despair concealed in her heart.

But I felt it. The next day Stephanie called me again and asked me about her situation.

'Can't wait to go back to school,' she told me in a low voice.

'Soon, you will be back at school.'

She arrested two days later. The team did all they could to save her but it was to no avail, as her heart was too weak. It was Sunday afternoon when she went to meet the Lord. Her dreams were all diminished. What a pity! For a few seconds I remained there, astounded, staring blankly at her lifeless body. I could not register the fact that only a day before I was talking to her, sharing her dreams and now it all perished with her.

She was gone now and there was only her memory which kept lingering within me. That was one of my first experiences, but death creates anguishing thoughts disturbing our realities. Yet, it is more hard when it hits young people, young souls.

The reality of our end dawns upon us unexpectedly when we least expected it. While we are young life appears eternal and the day of our final departure seems far away, buried in the distance of time. Suddenly, death appears like a thief in the night and robs our youth. Then we start asking questions, often without answers. Who am I? What is this journey? Death has become a common visitor in our ward and for me it was an unspoken journey which I dared not even delve into understanding.

Love was another journey which swept on me like a sweet dream. It helps to alleviate the pain and the somber reality afflicting me through my work.

The other side which was revealed to me was the beauty of love and it took me away from the environment with which I had to deal day by day. Ivan was handsome, tall with dark curly hair and pale skin.

That day we were short of staff and we could not work with few staff. Our Nurse in charge asked for more staff and Ivan was one of the extra staff who came to help us. My fate was inescapable and was already contriving my path before I even could dream it and while the dream presented itself to me, it was quite peculiar. Ivan was to be the dream, the guide to my course of life.

Often, I marvel at the trails of fate and when I look back I see this event as the initiation of episodes which led me to where I am now. Further on, the process lies in the journey and not the destination.

So he came in our ward, the wind touching my heart but he was also sculpting my statue. His name was Ivan and was a nurse. He approached me and asked me, 'Are you Francine?'

Our eyes met, his eyes were dark and penetrating and there was something in his voice which struck me. Yes, it conveyed me to another world which only belonged to our souls and it felt as though his voice transported me back in time, where there was only him and my soul to recall the beating of time spreading between us. This was rather a different emotion beating in my heart which differed to those which we face in our work.

I knew him but where? All I knew that my heart was racing. Was this love at first sight? Whatever this sentiment was, I was enjoying his company as it is quite rare that such handsome men cross my path during work. Ivan was very helpful and knew exactly what he was doing. The hours in the ward rolled by faster, like a dream, and work seemed lighter than usual and the gloomy feeling provoked by the apprehension of waiting for death ebbed away; at least for a while. Every time I was in his company I felt that twinge of reminiscence. Yes, his voice was the sound of so many years ago and it seemed that only my soul could recall the past. But I wanted to remain in the present, which seemed more attractive, promising me a dream which I wanted to live with in all my heart. Life was vibrating with a new a colour which I embraced heartily to alleviate the pain and sadness encountered in my work.

The following day I saw Ivan again in our ward. He approached me and told me that he had left his diary in our staffroom. But the diary was not in the staff room. Then before leaving he looked deeply into my eyes.

'Francine,' he uttered with his strong voice. 'Are you free tonight?'

I stared at him blankly, but feeling elated. I was speechless and could not find the proper words, the right words, for I tried to conceive if this was real or a beautiful dream which my mind was leading me to. I did not say anything, but he smiled at me and then said again, 'I would very much like to see you again. Can we meet tonight?'

I pondered and then I heard myself saying, 'Ok'

His eyes beamed and my heart fluttered.

'I'll see you tonight at Café Jubilee.'

So we agreed to meet that evening.

'I want to look into your eyes forever.' I heard him saying admiringly.

I felt elated, overpowered by these words, but could not say anything else.
I just smiled and looked into his eyes.
That was it. The journey of love has started for me for love comes when you least expect it and in that moment I knew that this man was going to reign over my heart for the days to come. In that moment in time, my life was being dictated by the beatings of my heart and I closed my eyes to follow its rhythm.

He walked out of the ward and I stood watching him. Rosanna, my colleague approached me.
'He's gorgeous.'
'Yes he is,' I muttered and walked away.
I went back to my work where an elderly patient was calling a nurse, so I went to help him. I felt jubilant, grasping the first breath of air and smiled to myself. This was a special day and I made sure I make most of it. It was a new horizon in the offering, but the journey was longer than I could have ever thought.

I often marvel at how a woman's perspective takes a different turn when she falls in love. The days appear shorter and the heart creates a wave of lightness that flows all over the body. This is what I was experiencing, like a wave of passion sweeping all over me, showering me with new emotions. There was a new beat in my heart which made me sweat and sent my blood rushing through my veins. It's an exhilarating experience which only the soul could comprehend and then engrave it in its memories.

SHATTERED WINGS

Café Jubilee is a popular cafe set in the heart of the city, quite close in the vicinities of the Court of Justice. This chic and small cafe offers a warm, friendly atmosphere and attracts a lot of people. Most of them work in court, or in business around the area, in this place anyone can discuss business, relax, or simply go there to have a good time. There is a touch of distinctive air which adds to the place's originality. Perhaps what makes it original is the amount of pictures hung all over the place, and various other ornaments which give a remarkable touch of originality; its unique style struck me. For instance, while looking up at the ceiling I could not help but marvel at the miniature table hung on the wall. Further along there was a miniature bike. At first glance it appeared rather strange, giving a different orientation to this place; yet, this innovative style did not interfere with the class and elegance of the place. It was a remarkable place to be in and especially now that I was waiting for the one who stole my heart.

Most of all, this place reminded one of an old brassiere or French Cabaret and combined with the warmth of the place one could conjure up many stories as well as escape from the harsh cold reality of everyday life. The pictures which were hung all over the walls were also interesting. Every picture depicted a particular theme related to that era. Overall, it was an amazingly creative place both for its construction and for its friendly atmosphere. This is what I thought while I waited impatiently for Ivan to come and meet me.

Impressed by the place, the dim light and warmth transported me back in time; I was enjoying picturing the most famous French artist Toulouse Lautrec. I visualized him in a similar cafe discussing art and his works with his Impressionists fellow artists. And the latter were most to my liking and their colours filled me with utter exultation, which swarmed all over my body. In this atmosphere my heart felt at peace. I ordered a cappuccino and went on reading extracts from the book which I have borrowed. The book was on the subject of Psychology, a topic which I liked, but that evening I was feeling somewhat overwhelmed, evoked by the beatings of my heart. The lines were too heavy for me, at least for that day and while I waited impatiently I just stared blankly at the pictures, magnificent in their originality and each disclosed a different story.

I was really enjoying traveling back in time, musing about the French era and visualising myself in that period, wearing a long red dress and attracting the attention of all. What fancies I was conjuring up, but then like someone in a dream I heard him uttering my name.
'Hi, Francine,' he said.
I looked up and saw him standing before me. Ivan appeared quite dashing, wearing a light blue shirt which really suited him and my heart started racing. Then he sat beside me and kissed me on my cheeks, looking at me closely.

His eyes permeated my soul and I felt the same thundering in my heart. This man was my dream.

SHATTERED WINGS

'You look beautiful,' he said with the same tenderness in his look which melted my heart. His sweet words were like a thousand drops of bliss caressing my heart. And in his company I felt like being born again away from the heavy burdens of the day. Tonight time had to stop, only for us and not even the attractive pictures could distract me now. His gaze took me into other decades, but most of all it took me through a journey within myself and in depths of my own emotions. I felt jubilant, lost in his gaze which was opening a new path for me. It was where I longed to be and I wished our encounter would remain forever. It lasted for a while.

We had dinner that night and we talked for long in the dim light of this romantic place looking into each other's eyes, the communication between us was even more heightened for our souls mingled and we could recall our existence in other eras. At least that was the feeling which I got in his presence, but what mattered was the present, the sweet moments of our hearts.

Above all, Ivan was a good listener with a sense of humor. With him I felt like an open book, as if I had known him for years. We could talk about everything, most of all about our work, and our aspirations.

Ivan was twenty five and was working in Malta for these last six months. He told me he had studied abroad and came to settle here. It was such a blessing, a sheer coincidence that we had to meet at this time. What I found most enchanting in Ivan was the fact that he was interesting and with him I could talk about practically everything.

The night which followed that day was going to remain engraved in my heart, as if seeds were planted in me, which were to be of absolute significance for me, most of all for my heart. Instinctively, I knew that I was not going to remain the same, as my heart in the stillness of that magical night had weaved its path. The steps of my heart were determined, but I was still in the hands of fate; the same fate which ordained the struggle between life and death for my patients. It was now ordering mine.

Providence had to decree that we continue this dream. And indeed it did.

So, it appeared that our destinies decided to bring us together, and that our meetings should continue. That was until the holder of our destinies decided to intervene, but until that day I kept moving with the waves presented before me, which I had to embrace and enclose with the petals of my heart. And so I did, letting myself dance with the rhythm of my heart, writing a poem contrived of pure sentiments for the man who presented himself in this new journey, this dream. The more I thought of Ivan, the more I longed to be with him. And so our encounters went on.
There was no doubt that I was in love with him and that my feet throbbed on the path prepared by fate. Each breath changed me, changed my life and

every time I looked at the sky my thoughts would transport me into another world, another heart. A bridge of light to his heart, and it felt like a burning fire taking over me.

The days went by and I could not imagine myself living without Ivan. He was all I could ask for, a loving and understanding man. It was what I wanted in love and for a while I thought I attained it.

And while this beautiful dream flourished, I went on. Months flew on, which brought new life for me, it felt like a new birth as I threaded the path of love or I fathomed to be so.

Yet, nothing stays the same, no matter how we seek to control our lives. Soon it was time for my dream to take a different turn and then one fine day Ivan spoke about his sister and that was the first path of unveiling the truth. The truth! I wonder for how long a woman can dream in her heart and let herself be led into a deep sea of emotions without opening her eyes. Perhaps, it is a talent letting our souls travel into abyss of illusions, till truth can not stand any longer hidden behind veils. And this was the birth of a new phase…another journey, but life is all small trips which opens doorways to oneself.

The sea, with its crystal hues, is the reflection of the soul, but it is also the keeper of many secrets. The sun was sitting warmly on the horizon, casting its blazing fire on the waves of love which then faded bit by bit. We were emerging from the cold days of the gloomy winter and the waves were calm as if welcoming the new season.

I was there with Ivan, as we often visited the sea; it was our refuge and escape from our daily life, where we could get lost in each other's arms leading to our hearts. It was where we could express our passions and breathe of life in all its beauty. Life was a genuine promise, taking me away from scenes of its departure in my work. But here I had to forget and concentrate on the throbbing pulses of that heart close to mine. Life was indeed beautiful! I thought as I touched the harsh palms, yet soft and caressed with the popular sentiment which we both knew in our hearts.

We sat on a rock facing the horizon and I could only hope that our horizon would not ebb away, but remain engraved on our fates. Ivan looked deeply into my eyes and my heart leaped with joy. A strange wave of passion took over me as he spoke with his gentle voice.
'Francine,' he was saying, 'Since, I met you my life has changed and I will never ever leave you.'
Sweet words which could melt the hardest rock, but when I look back I admonish myself for my naivety. I had been an innocent girl taken by the luring words of the wind waiting to deceive me. Yet, as long as my eyes were closed I lived in this contrived path. Then it was too late.
I smiled and kissed him on his cheeks.
'Mine too,' I uttered.
'I love you Francine, you are my life'.

SHATTERED WINGS

These are poetic words which every woman long to hear. So, I chose that night to immerse myself in his sweet words which were like waves of a poem opening up fresh petals in my heart.
'I love you,' he repeated.
'I love you too,' I said feeling the passion travelling all over my body urging me to become closer and unite with the man I loved.

If there was something being concocted I could not see it, as it was well conceited. In Ivan's company I only felt complete happiness, and my heart was opened to him. That evening was magical, but there was something different, however I could not see it. For me there was only him, my beloved.

I kissed him on his lips without making any effort to restrain the passions which flooded all over my body. There was fire burning in all parts of my body and I wanted to taste the beauty of love which comes like crystal water falls. It was pure love and I let myself go with its flow. While we embraced the waves, which danced deep within us, I felt elated, lost in the sea of emotions and passion. The sun had set and it was darker, the loving spirits of the stars appeared to watch over us, sent from the God to protect our love. That is what I hoped, and after the sweet communication of our bodies, it was time to speak with our minds.

Ivan spoke about his sister who lived in Italy. His gaze was suddenly serious. This must be really worrying him. He was saying something.
'Francine, I am really worried.'

'I know that, my love,' I uttered as I fondled his hair. He looked at me with those warm penetrating eyes. 'My sister called me the other day and told me that she is having problems with her husband.'

'Oh, I am really, sorry,' I heard myself saying.

But why was he talking about his sister? Why, in such a magical place secluded only for us and for our love and bliss. Yet, behind those words there was another story which was slowly, slowly carving my own life.

Ivan was adamant in keeping with the subject and this seemed to be on his mind for he mentioned her again.

'It was a shock for us. They were perfect together.'

Genuinely, I felt sorry for them for it was such a pity to lose the magic and sweetness of love. Little did I know that this reality was going to be my next path, where the Nymph of love suddenly becomes the Medusa.

'I hope that we do not go through that experience.' it was all I could say.

He stroked my cheeks with his soft large palms.

Silence stood between us and for a moment, neither of us uttered any single word. I stared at the waves, moving swiftly, embracing the stillness of the day contrary to my heart. Now, there was no stillness, but a shadow of doubt which I tried not to heed. I looked again at Ivan. He too was staring at the sea. Was he thinking of our future? Or was it something else which I could not yet apprehend.

SHATTERED WINGS

I felt a lump in my throat. Instantly, I decided to cancel the thought from my mind and instead I caressed the wavy hair of my beloved, hoping to instill the peace which was disturbed by this single thought. Yet, when I look back I think differently and today I claim that this was the beginning of my end. In that moment I was blinded by love. Ivan looked at me and his eyes were smiling again. The magic of the sea, I thought. I sighed with relief and caressed his hands. He then spoke again.

'Next week, my cousin, Salvatore will be coming and we will be discussing the situation.'

'Fine,' I said.

So, he was still thinking about his sister's situation. But why all this endless thoughts and concerns for his sister, when I was beside him? People love each other and then anything can happen, but I did not want it to happen to me. No, never.

Ivan stroked my hands and we were surrounded again by deep silence which reigned between us and even the soft sound of the waves was fading. The waves were conveying a message which was hard to grasp. Then Ivan spoke again, 'Let's forget about it, we will never go through that experience I promise. His words were comforting, but my thoughts were overshadowed by a concept which I could not understand. It was yet to be unfolded on the clouds of fate.

He looked into my eyes and said tenderly, 'Your eyes are shining.'

'It's because they are looking at you.'

He smiled and kissed me.
'I love you, you cannot imagine how much.'
I smiled and the waves peered hideously at me.
Was it sharing the same sentiment?

There was a dream which disturbed me, even
though I rarely doted on dreams, but this was quite
different from the others. In the dream I saw Ivan
standing alone in the gallery. A familiar voice called
me.
'Francine, Francine.'
I looked back and followed the voice. I followed the
voice and came face to face with one of the young
patients I most loved. Stephanie. She was all clad
in white and her eyes were like quartz crystals.
'Francine,' she said, 'Ivan is married.' Married! Her
voice echoed in the distance. I woke up startled,
her words still hammering in my ears. But why did
this dream come to torment me? There was a
theory that at times the departed from us appear in
dreams to warn us. But was there any warning?
No, Stephanie could not be aware of this. So I
banished the dream from my memory.

Then the dream came to haunt me in reality. I met
Salvatore, Ivan's cousin, two days later and I
instantly felt at ease with him. Salvatore was rather
was tall, dark and in his early forties, but with a
particular charm so prevalent among the Italians.
There was no resemblance with Ivan, perhaps
because he was older. Yet, Salvatore still retained
his looks; I guessed he had been really handsome
when younger. Just like Ivan.

SHATTERED WINGS

One afternoon, in the glorious days of spring, we met in a cafe and Ivan introduced me to his cousin. Salvatore was separated from his wife and lived in Italy, in Milan, where he worked as an electrical engineer and was staying for some time in Malta. He said he had some business to attend to. Coming from the warmth of the Mediterranean, Salvatore was similar to us, talkative, open and friendly. We immediately felt comfortable in each other's company and for me this was an opportunity to practice the Italian language. That made it easier for him and we could talk about everything under the sun, but mainly we talked about work and about Italy. Unaware of the real purpose for his visit I found myself enchanted by Salvatore. If only I'd known the purpose of his visit, then I would not be writing these lines.

Weeks flew rapidly and the days faded with the clouds; with every new day my love for Ivan increased and my heart was completely open for him. Ivan became the center of my life. Work and my other aspirations had taken second place in my life. Now, he was my life. Looking back, I say it was not right; I had been misled by the games of love. Yet, at that time I felt elated, living in a world which I have conjured up. There was a sweet dream lingering in my soul. Someone had to stop this dream, and this someone had to be Salvatore, as this incident was already inscribed in my book of fate. This was an incredible, revolting truth which demolished every hope I could have had.

For reasons which I thought were related to business, Salvatore decided to prolong his visit in Malta for more days. Ivan was happy about this for they could spend more time together; or so they led me to believe. But Salvatore's visit on the island had nothing to do with business. It was to do with me, or better with my love. It was like thunderbolt, but I had to go through it. The day was cold and cloudy and it descended upon me like unexpected rain. I shall never forget the day when my eyes were at last opened to witness the truth. And in this act, Salvatore, the charming cousin was chosen to deliver the message, to unveil the truth which changed my life and gave it a different direction.

I have no idea if he felt this burden, but I often marvel at how others were contriving in my path without my knowing. What I thought belonged to me in one moment in time was taken way by the by the next one. It is rather strange how fate can suddenly decide to alter one's path, overnight! All of a sudden, without any warning or any hinge of what was coming, my towers tumbled down upon me and left me destitute, shattered by the wings of fate. And it was on one particular day. Dawn came as usual to give birth to the womb of earth. It came also for me, descending on my chart of life. That evening I had to meet Ivan and Salvatore in the usual cafe, enjoying its typical warm atmosphere. I went into the cafe and looked for Salvatore. He was sitting alone smoking a cigar and drinking an espresso. As soon as he saw me he waved and I approached him. Salvatore kissed me on both cheeks, as was traditional.

SHATTERED WINGS

'Hi Salvatore,' I said and sat down beside him hoping that Ivan would come soon.
'Cara, how are you?' he asked smiling.
'I'm fine thank you, and you?'
'Fine,' he said looking directly into my eyes.

All at once there was silence between us. I hate silence; it gives way for other thoughts to be formed. Yes, we were dominated by a strange silence which I could not comprehend; yet, my heart was pounding, like endless beatings of drums, hammering and hammering till there was no space left, until my heart could understand the underlying meaning on the pattern of fate. It was fate which defeated me and from the onset of my days was preparing a path.

Salvatore was speechless for most of the time, which was rather unusual for him. By nature he was talkative, but today he seemed pensive. Something must have happened. I thought.
I had this strange inkling, that it was something which concerned Ivan.
To my relief, Salvatore broke the silence.
'I am finding Malta a very nice country.'
'It pleases me to hear that.' I retorted.

To keep the conversation going I asked him if he had been to the Temples, my favourite spot, my refuge where I managed to communicate with time. It had been quite a long time since I visited them. How I longed to go there now!
Salvatore spoke again

'I must visit the temples. A friend of mine told me the Temples are very interesting.'
'Indeed,' I replied, 'the giant temples are constructed in conjunction with the sun and constellation.'

He was smiling, 'Francine, you really amuse me, and at times I envy my cousin.'
I was taken aback by his words and thought that his statement was rather sardonic, so I spoke again, changing the subject.
'My friends told me Italy is very nice.'
'Indeed it is. And have you been to Italy?'
'No, but I'd love to go some time.'
He then smoked a cigarette.
'You must come to Italy for some time.'
He paused and then looked at me again gazing in my eyes. His gaze annoyed me, but I tried to ignore it.

'Should you decide to come, let me know and I will show you around.'
'Thanks,' I said, 'Perhaps, yes I will visit Italy with Ivan, though it depends on our work.'
'Of course,' he continued. 'You work very hard.'
'It's a demanding job. Thank God that we work in the same department, so we can meet very often.'

Salvatore looked at me thoughtfully and did not utter any single word.
My mind was lost in a train of thoughts, I was wondering where Ivan had got to. Three quarters of an hour have elapsed and he had not turned up. Meanwhile my conversation with Salvatore was

becoming rather strange. I kept talking to him, looking forward to seeing the man of my dreams, ruler of my heart.

He did not turn up and being away from him I was getting this sense of foreboding feeling that something must have happened to him. It was rather unusual for Ivan to arrive late. Salvatore went on talking about Italy and his work and time on the island and the conversation was becoming rather stale. My mind was whirling, wondering what could have happened to Ivan. Time went by and he still did not appear. I was becoming frantic and overwhelmed by these thoughts. Something must have happened.

As if in answer to all these thoughts and doubts, the cell phone rang. It was Ivan. I sighed with relief. He told me he was in Sliema waiting for us in a Restaurant. I could only thank God that he was safe and sound. My love was waiting on the other side and my agonizing thoughts vanished.

This was only for a while. Salvatore offered to take me to Sliema where we were to meet, and I accepted. Salvatore was driving the car and was talking all the way, but that was only prompting me to overlook reality.

'I got used to your way of driving now. To be honest it was not easy.'

'I know, we drive on the right.'

Salvatore then looked at me.

'So for how long have you been going out with my cousin?'

'Almost six months,' I affirmed.
'Hmm,' I heard him say, but then kept driving.

It did not take me long to realise that he was not taking me to Sliema, and for some reason, which I could not conceive, he took a different turn. It was not to Sliema. Could it be he'd lost his way? Sliema was quite an easy destination to reach, which by now he was familiar with. We were supposed to meet Ivan at eight o'clock, but it was quarter past now. Then it occurred to me that we were not heading to our destination. Salvatore was not taking me there. But what was the reason behind this? What intentions could he have? No, I was conjuring things up, letting my fanciful mind take over. My longing to see Ivan took over me. But I had been warned.
'Salvatore, where are you taking me?' I asked him.
Then I was to know for he replied.
'We will soon be there, but I know a better place where we can be alone together.'
Alone together! The words echoed in my mind. What was he saying? His words were rather confounding and I did not understand what he had in mind. Alone together, he said. Why? For a moment I thought I pertained to another world, another reality.
'Salvatore,' I insisted, 'I want to meet Ivan.'
'Ivan? You said Ivan.'
'Yes,' I replied.

Salvatore looked at me and laughed. His smile made me feel uneasy and my stomach churned. No, I could not comprehend what have taken over him. Instead he drove towards the direction of Manoel Island which is a remote solitary area. It is normally used for yachts and no one goes there late. I shuddered and my feet felt clammy, he was contriving something which I could not infer to.

'Stop Salvatore,' I cried.
He kept on driving further into the place which I dreaded.
'Why my dear?' he asked with a sardonic smile on his lips.

My God! I was distraught, what could I do? Now, I was certain that he was not taking me to Ivan. He parked his car in a remote corner facing the boats. Not one single soul could be seen, nor any single animal. The blood rushed in all over my veins, but there was another terror which I could not detect.

'Salvatore, take me to Ivan,' I pleaded almost sobbing and with trepidation running all over my veins.
'Why, my beauty? Why don't you listen to me? '

This was unacceptable and he gave me no time, not even to utter any single word for he moved close to me. Then he brought his lips close to mine. My heart quivered and I was breathless, invaded by his odor of cigarettes and alcohol. This was a bad dream, yet his ardent imposed kisses reaffirmed that this was indeed reality. Someone else was kissing my lips and this someone was not Ivan. My soul had been invaded by someone whom I never expected. I managed to release myself.

'No Salvatore.'

He was taken aback and then continued 'I cannot resist you, you drive me crazy.'

'Salvatore, please would you take me to Ivan?' I cried.

'Ivan?' he said laughingly, 'Forget about him.'

'No, he is the man of my heart and, I love him,' I said tenderly.

'Then, my dear you love the wrong man. Ivan is does not belong to you. He is married.'

His words struck me like thunder. I stared at him, disbelieving what he was implying.

'What are you saying? You must be out of your mind.'

I thought that was one of his motives to win my affections and make me succumb to his passions. I could only hope.

'No, Francine,' he continued, 'I have no intention to lie to you, Ivan is married to my cousin. I brought you here to tell you the truth. He wanted me to meet you as he thought we would get together.'

A chill ran up and down my spine. How could he use this lie? No, he was lying. Then, I plucked up the courage and slapped him on his cheeks.

'Liar,' I cried.

He blushed and lowered his head.

'Now let me go,' I yelled.

He seized me again, 'Not before I tell you everything. That I like you, I cannot hide it, but I have no intentions to conceal the truth from you. Ivan is married to my cousin Marisa; she is not his sister, but his wife.'

SHATTERED WINGS

His sister and not his wife! His words hammered in my ears and I felt like blades piercing me bit by bit. My thoughts traveled back to that day, watching the sunset with Ivan. I could still see his gaze, but why did he conceal it if it was real? No wonder I had that feeling.

'I want to see him now,' I retorted.

'Ivan should be in Italy right now.'

How could this be? Some minutes away he had called me.

'No, it cannot be. Ivan called me to meet him.' I told him.

Salvatore spoke again.

'Francine, I am sorry for you. Ivan is in Rome and he was calling us from there.'

His words pierced my heart like daggers. Was this a dream? I stared at him, but I could not believe him. Ivan, the man I adored, the one who ruled my heart belonged to someone else. Once he was my dream and now he was my executioner, for he betrayed me. He deceived me, he let me love him. Tears were rolling down on my cheeks and a lump in my throat almost felt like choking me.

Salvatore stroked my hair. 'Poor Francine, I can see that you love him, but he cannot return your love, you are wasting your time, you are so beautiful.'

Salvatore's words did not console me, I was feeling rejected by the man whom I thought loved me. There was no other way. My walls crushed upon me. Then, Salvatore tried to kiss me again, but I managed to get away from him and got out of the car. I walked as fast as I could away from his car.

I was in a trance, and if it was not for my feet which led me out of the place I would not get out of this isolated area which I detested. My mind was overwhelmed, overpowered by this shattering truth which besieged me when I was expecting the beauty of love to unfold. Instead there were torn petals of abstruse truth.

It was dark in my room and night fell upon my soul like a bird with tattered wings. These were my wings which were taken by this shattering reality which was suffocating me. Yet, I was still hoping that it was not so. That night I lay restless, overtaken by shock. With this devastating reality haunting me, I kept seeing his face, his sweet words, of our love when it was all lies and betrayal and that was closer. I wanted it, I longed for it. Salvatore's words kept lingering in my mind. Could he have a secret agenda? He wanted me for himself, maybe he was lying and wanted to come between us; I could only hope.

Yet, an inner voice deep within me confirmed that Salvatore's words were a mere mirror of facts.
Suddenly, I recalled that strange dream. It was no strange dream, but a premonition of reality.
Love with its splendour and evergreen dreams had deserted me and left me naked in the wind.
The journey was over; it vanished with the waves which made me dream once.

SHATTERED WINGS

I returned to work and the ward looked bleak and dark, as if I was being transported into a tunnel of darkness. I could not cope with the everyday pains. My thoughts were constantly about Ivan, but I wanted to hear the truth from his mouth. My love could not do that to me, to my heart. Where was the poem near the sea? And the crystal love in our eyes?

It all perished in one night, which only came to rob my peace, like a thief in the night it came to stifle the fire which was blazing in my heart. Now it was cold, freezing more than snow and I knew that it was going to remain like this for the days to come. Again my work had become the centre of my life. Ivan had to be concealed forever from my mind. But I was embarking on an impossible   trip.

The hours slipped away and there was a lot of work which helped me to alleviate my troubles. The day went on and during the break I decided to call him. My hands were trembling and the answering voice echoed, emerging from within. Ivan was on leave, abroad and this verified the facts which I have heard from his cousin. My thoughts were shaken and there was no denying now, I have let myself be beguiled by the mask of love.

The truth dawned upon me and showered me with tiny drops. It was a windy day, the wind, blowing hard, entered from one of the windows in the ward. It felt like tearing my heart into thousand petals, devastated by the shattering winds of fate. And now it all changed! Gone were the days when I kissed those lips under the setting sun. At this moment his lips were kissing some one else, yet I could not register it. My heart longed to hear the truth being uttered by his sweet lips, which now turned into a cynical kiss.

A month passed by, and every new day was like threading on passages of Hell and it was only through my work that I found comfort. Then one day the wind brought him back. I was at work when he called me. My heart stopped beating and shivers ran all over my spine. His voice steered inside me, arousing the same ways of passion. I could not deny it, I still loved him.

'How are you my love?' I heard him say.

'I am fine.' I said firmly.

'Francine, I want to see you before I go back again,' he went on.

'There is nothing more to say,' I said.

'We need to talk,' he insisted.

He wanted to face me now, to discuss things, perhaps. I could not face him, not after his treacherous plan to hide the truth away from me. But what did he want from me? What all men want from women, an inner voice warned me. That was it. There was nothing more to say now that things had to be settled between us. Yet, I agreed to meet him, perhaps for the last time. A strange feeling propelled me to accept. Yes, for the last time, even though I felt confounded, lost in a sea of mixed emotions, buried in the echo of love.

SHATTERED WINGS

Indeed, love was still in my heart, when all he did was betray me with another woman, who in sheer reality was his wife. He now belonged to her.

And all the time he knew about it.

The next day I headed for the Upper Barracca where we had to meet. The Upper Barracca is large garden with a large balcony facing the Grand Harbour. This is a rather romantic place enriched with the foreshadowing remnants of history. For years it had witnessed battles, bloodshed and finally victory over its enemies and most people enjoy going there to admire the great Fortresses which once struggled to protect the city. The fortresses were stronger than I was; a cold wave of helplessness took over me, rendering me vulnerable to fates games. I felt lost, but above all I had lost and my battle was lost. Long endless silence reigned in this place, but there was no silence now in my heart, only long tormenting thoughts which manifested themselves into pain. The day was warm with the sun bestowing its rays on the building, typical of a September day, which when hitting all the building it created a remarkable picturesque scene.

Not for me. My heart felt heavy thrown into deep isolation. I yearned for the old days when I was exuberant, laughing at life. Where was that girl? That girl was now immersed in the wilderness, where only tears exist. These were the thoughts which accompanied the tears which rolled down my cheeks while I waited.

Ivan appeared, entering the gardens looking very handsome, but in my vision he looked more handsome, probably because I knew I was losing him. Strange I pondered, some months before he was the reason for living.

Ivan approached me.
'How are you?' he said.
'I'm fine,' I heard myself saying.
I looked into his eyes, dark and beaming. How many times did I peer into them while imaging them as the sea of love and passion? Today they were cold and aloof, unveiling the deceit which he contrived in his heart. He sat beside me and my heart was beating faster. Then, Ivan took my hands and started caressing them. A shiver ran all over my spine, but I had to confront reality.

I decided to start the conversation and go straight to the point.
'Ivan,' I began by saying, 'You lied to me, you did not tell me that you were married.'
He did not show any emotion but stared at me not even uttering a single word.
'Ivan,' I repeated, 'Tell me it's not true, tell me.'
Again, he did not answer, but instead Ivan turned his head to the other direction.
Silence stood between us, cutting my heart like a knife. The air felt stifling and I knew what to conjecture as this devastating truth was knocking at my heart. He then broke the silence which was almost killing me and shedding me into pieces.

SHATTERED WINGS

'Francine, I am married, but I loved you. I could not tell you.'

I felt a lump in my throat, tears flooding in my eyes while my stomach ached. This was the truth emerging from his lips. The lips I longed to kiss, even now while I was facing this treacherous situation. My heart still longed to break this barrier between us and to lure him back.

There was nothing and Ivan's words brought me to reality.

'My wife is Italian, and Salvatore is her cousin. Francine, please try to understand me, I loved you and I did not want to leave you.'

Hearing the truth coming from his mouth was painful and it tore my heart into pieces. There was no way out of this puzzle. Could I believe him?

'You could have told me. Ivan you lured me into loving you when all the time you were tied to someone else. How could you?' I sobbed.

'You're right, yes by that time we were not together, then I met you and I fell in love with you.'

Fall in love, he said? How could he be so beguiling, falling in love with an innocent woman when he was married?

How dared he call this love? For me it was love, for I was ready to give my life for him. Now he has taken my dreams. He lowered his head and did not say another word. I couldn't speak, nor look at him again.

Then I found the courage and said, 'You used me Ivan.'

A surge of rage took over me and propelled me to act. I slapped him on his cheeks. He looked at me, startled. Tension was stronger between us and he spoke again 'No, Francine, I loved you and I still do.'

Could I trust him now? No, my vision was blurred and I felt like a destructed tower. I wanted to yell, to scratch his face, to beat him, but the sheer devastating thought residing deep inside me was more painful. I still loved this man and this made it harder.
'What are you doing now?' I asked him.
'I will be settling in Italy.'
'Then go to Hell.'
'No Francine.'

So that was it. No other solution could solve this riddle. I got up and hurriedly I walked out of the place. Ivan did not belong to me any longer; foolishly I let him take over my heart which he misused. These are lessons, part of the journey called love which for me ended abruptly. There were more to come and silence was my only solace, for this experience was soon buried deep within me. Yet, the pain was hard to bear as it was engraved in my heart. But fight I would, I was still young and I had to move on. There was still my work, my mission, where the patients could not wait for long and they needed my help and my courage, even though in my heart I was not feeling it. Nonetheless, this tragedy I was there for them. And that was what kept me going which helped to instill a new inner peace.

SHATTERED WINGS

For most of the time I cried, also to relieve myself from the pain and void created by Ivan. He was a dream which touched me for a short moment and then flew away, leaving me speechless, exposed and awestruck.

He was my first love and would always be. But what were these candid thoughts? He left a week after our encounter. Better for me, and I hoped that he would be happy with his family, for deep within my heart I felt that was the path of true love, wishing the best for the one you love, even if you had to let him go.

Prostrated with grief as I was, my flame of love had to be put out. I was determined to keep on going, to revert back to the old Francine, the cheerful girl who smiled at life. I met other men and amongst them was James, a handsome teacher. James was interesting and in his company I felt good. It helped to alleviate the heartbreaking pain caused by Ivan. His memory was fading, but every new dawn reminded me of him, and deep within me I reckoned that I never ceased to love him and he was forever inscribed in my heart.

They say time is the best healer. Yes, the thought of him created tears, but there were other horizons waiting for me. Life flowed with its ups and downs. I have changed and learnt a lot from my experience, the disappointment opened up a new path for me and through these revelations I gained inner strength.

Strangely, another voyage was unfolding, bringing new lessons. Men were there to present conflicts, perhaps lessons which can be sweet as honey and harsh as stone.

It is the waves of fate created by time or by our soul.

Juan was ten years old when he was admitted in our ward for treatment. It was all to no avail as he was diagnosed with the fatal illness of Leukemia and there was little chance of recovery. Professor Borg did all he could to save the boy, but it was evident he was not going to live.
It was such a pity to see such a young boy in such misery, but this was part of our everyday reality, a part which I would never get used to.

Juan was a charming young boy, but he was cast down by a curse, which threatened his days. He could not plan for the future for it was already planned for him like all of us. Each of us follow this plan and Juan's plan was to leave this world at an early age just when he should be starting life.
I liked to talk with him and he liked to talk about his father and of the limited time they had together.
'My father is an influential man on the island,' he said one day.
'You must be very proud,' I retorted.

I could see the freckles of light in his eyes when he talked about his father. He was very fond of him, an only child in the family. I liked to sit beside his bedside and listen to him while he talked about his dear father, yet the destructive wave of death was standing at the door waiting for the right moment. It must be a big blow for them, his father being such an important man. If only I could stop these waves from entering and taking away the innocent souls and the fresh petals of youth. I thought. Instinctively, Juan knew, he would be traveling to the other world and the only solace was the thought of his successful father.

I met his father two days later. He was a politician, a Member of Parliament. George was a tall man in his late forties and one afternoon while he was visiting his son, he approached me.

'Miss, I really appreciate what you are doing for my son.' he started by saying.

I gazed at his dark eyes under his curly hair which was turning grey. He was handsome and I could easily see that Juan has taken his looks.

'Sorry, but you are..?' I asked politely.

'I'm George, Juan's father.'

We shook hands. The man was very smart, but was warm. It was the first time I had met a politician. They always gave me the impression of being distant and aloof, but this man was another version far different from the impression which I conjured up in my thoughts.

'We are doing all we can,' was all I could say.

'I know and I am really grateful. It is very hard to accept that our only son is leaving us.'

He lowered his head. He was pondering on the sheer reality which befall him. And I thought that death has no boundaries and was the only equilibrium in life. Juan s' father was very powerful,

perhaps more than we could see, yet, he could not conquer death.
He was losing the battle like all of us.

'I understand, well, we try to make his last days easy,' I added.
'God will reward you, Ms Francine.'
'It's my duty,' I said humbly.
'Yours is a mission, it shows in your eyes.'
'Thanks, now I must go,' I said feeling rather embarrassed by his remark, so I left him alone in the corridor.

It was a quite a hard task to address the patients' relatives being aware that there was no hope. If only I knew what was awaiting me. Juan went to the other dimension a week after. I was there until the last moment, till the last breath, witnessing the departure of this angel.

I saw his parents' faces turning ghastly pale as he uttered his last words, and that was the end for Juan, but the beginning of another journey for me.

Days continued passing swiftly and with each day I drifted away from my past. Ivan was only a memory and I engulfed myself completely in my work, focusing my attention of my patients. It was now time for another lesson and some months after Juan passed away I got a mysterious phone call. I was in the ward with a patient when I was told there was a call for me. I went to answer the phone. It was a man's voice. My heart throbbed and I felt the blood rushing to my veins. My head felt suddenly heavy as I thought he was Ivan.

Why now?

To my relief it was not him, but I was heading for another incredulous phase which hit me deeply and rested with me for the days which followed.
This was another baffling situation, which was destined to leave its mark forever in my life. And it was more traumatic than losing love. This was a scar or better a grave wound which never healed.
'How can I help you?' I said in a formal voice.
And it was George, Juan's father who spoke.
'How are you Francine?' he asked me with his warm voice, yet at the same time demanding authority.
'I'm ok,' I replied unaware of what was to come.
'For me life is a struggle, you know after Juan's death.'
'I fully understand, but have faith.' I tried to comfort him.
'Francine, you are beautiful, I like you.'

His words astounded me and for a moment I thought I was hearing someone else. But no, it was George who was saying these strange words. His sentence was out of context and not appropriate.
'Good day, Mr. George,' I said firmly, 'I must leave you, if you do not mind.'
But he persisted in an annoying way.
'No dear, I thought, you and I would meet one day. What do you think?'
'No, it can never be,' I said firmly.

His words disturbed me and left me speechless. It seems to me that he did not take my message..
'Dear Francine, I loved you from the very first time I saw you.'
'I do not care,' I affirmed and cut the line.

For a moment I stared at the phone, disbelieving my ears. How could this be? To me it sounded rather strange and this was another nightmare. I tried to ignore the fact and went on with my work. My mind was overwhelmed with thoughts about that unexpected telephone call.
Within an hour he called me again.
'Leave me alone,' I said.
'I can't leave you, I want you and will not leave you until I get what I want,' he insisted.
'Then it is really your problem,' I responded boldly, 'it would be better if you leave me alone, even for you.'

This situation left me bewildered and I was at loss. Why did he have to call? Had I been too friendly with him? Then I reassured myself that it was not so. This relieved me for a while. Or maybe I thought so. And these were the thoughts which accompanied me. He called me again, but I could not answer. Then he stopped and I felt relieved for I could continue with my work. Days rolled by faster like the others, each day took me away from all the previous events. I was even smiling again, but this was only for a short while when the veils of illusion were lifted. Precisely when I thought that I got rid of George, the past he appeared again. This time he came strongly leaving his mark, a wound which could never heal.

This inner peace which I strived so hard to have was not written in my path, and after the devastating experience another one was unfolding. It appeared to me that my life had to be perturbed by these endless events which threw me into a whirlwind of confusion and attempted to drown me into a sea of utter loneliness. I was sharing the drama faced by our patients. Another deadly event was approaching and one which altered my direction in life. There were more days to come, but one day had a different impact for me and was going to remain with me for eternity. That day invaded me and no night, no day, any sun or moon can alleviate the thundering storm which this day left in my heart.

Yes, another bleak day dawned upon me. I wished that day never gave birth to daybreak. Then I longed to go back in time, even if possible to the moments I spent with Ivan. Ivan betrayed me, but his treason tasted sweeter when compared with the bitterness of what I had to go through. It only instilled revenge and more anger. The time when love betrayed me appeared in that moment more secure. If only I could go back and remain looking at the waves. But I could not even if I wanted to.

I was expecting that night to be joyful; I was expecting a night away from pain and sadness of my everyday life. I went out with my friends where we went to a disco and for a moment I felt being relieved from the past and every step seemed to bring me back freedom. The music took me out of myself, and I untied all the chains which bound me.

Just for a while, that night deceived me too. Its purpose was to give birth to an experience aiming to take me away from bliss and dancing. I was introduced to a nightmare which then kept on visiting me in my bad dreams. In the darkness of night I was raped, invaded by an outsider who was not a complete outsider. It is not till one goes through the experience that one starts to comprehend the real meaning of this crime, the sin of men.

That night was dedicated to them.

It was time for us to go and one of my friends drove me home. It was barely midnight, but we were working on the next day so Sarah, dropped me in the vicinities of my residence. I only had five minutes walk to reach home. Suddenly I realised that I was not alone, there was someone walking behind me. It did not matter until they started to come closer and now their presence was imminent, so close that I could even smell their scent.

I looked back and was stupefied to see the appalling figure of George standing there. A cold shiver ran all over my spine and the blood in my veins had turned cold. Yet, another bad dream and could not be reality, I thought. He stood there, but I was not going to let him intimidate me.

SHATTERED WINGS

I plucked up the courage and asked him, 'What do you want?'
He did not answer.

Deep silence was his answer, but I knew that he was up to something. At once I thought of his calls and my feet turned suddenly cold and I was sweating. I made an effort to run away, but he was swifter than me. George grabbed my hands and threw on the ground. I got up quickly and started running, but like a ferocious animal he was there holding me tightly. He forced me inside his car which was not far away and locked the door and then drove away.

I had not the slightest idea for where he was heading and dejection took over me. This was a trap and I was his prey.
'Leave me,' I cried.
My cry was to no avail for his mind was already set. George knew what he wanted to do, far before this event.
'I won't. You know want I want from you.'
'I do not care what you want,' I shouted.

I could only hope that he would change his direction but I was wrong, very wrong. George stopped the car in a far away corner and then the worst was yet, to come for his body was already upon mine. I felt breathless as he forcefully grasped my chest tearing my top. He kissed my lips while his left hand pressed my breasts. Then he came closer, his breath smelling of pungent alcohol, was suffocating me. It felt like being invaded by a vicious animal which I could not resist. He then took off my skirt and I could do nothing. His hands moved swiftly all over my breasts, pressing them hard to the point of hurting me badly. I cried, but he covered my mouth and with the other hand he moved towards my thighs, tearing my underwear. With his harsh hands he moved towards my private part and his hard touch was painful. It was a sharp pain and it felt like scissors entering deep within me tearing every part of me.

I cried and cried, but this seemed to accelerate his lust. The worst was yet to come for he made an attempt to force his body closer. It felt hard and the only protection was to tighten my thighs, but this made it harder. A hard piece of wood was being enforced, entering between my thighs. No matter how I resisted, but he kept moving fiercely and thrusting himself inside of me. It was hard and created an intense pain like a dagger inside my inner velvet.

I could not bear the sharp intense pain, which by now was increasing. I thought I was going to die, but I did not, instead there was more pain, points of daggers tearing me inside out and then it felt moist like a flow of swarming liquid moving from him deep within me. He took a deep breath and yelled, but I almost fainted.

I closed my eyes. I had been deflowered, this was my first time. The sharp pain was now transported to my heart. I did not even do it with Ivan, the only man I loved. Not even during our warmest kisses near the sea.

Where was that passion now?

It all perished as if it never existed. I did not want to think of passion now, only of this savage all over my body. This savage was taking from me something which he did not deserve and I detested him. His fierce movements planted in my cells; a new seed that of revenge.

There were no tears, even if tears would relieve me from this hell, they deserted me and left me alone to face the pain. Where was I? Yes, I was floating on water, but it was painful, very painful. As if they have set fire in the lower part of my body. It was destroying me, soon this fire will take all over and then I will leave this body.

He was sweating and panting breathlessly. I was disgusted by him and every man on this earth. Yet, there was nothing I could do. I heard him utter some words. I guessed these were some filthy words which were not to my understanding, but still it was shameful and I felt dead. He was killing me, his hideous thing felt like a hot poker inside me. My velvet was destroyed and burning with pain. He then kissed me again, his lips tasted like poison, then his fingers moved again. I felt rotten now. Then he touched my thighs, I felt speechless, lost in another world. My spirit has gone somewhere else and I did not belong here.

The woman in the car was a puppet, but the words he uttered were sharp which I could clearly understand.

'Francine, you taunted me, you led me into this, remember, I am an important man, don't you dare open your mouth. Now go.'

He took a deep breath and then I heard him say, 'My dear, I can still smell your petals.'

'Bastard!' I heard myself saying, and slapped him on his face, but I knew that I was going to remember this horrid night for all my life. He unlocked the door of the car and I got out of it. I laid on the ground and cried. Where was I? I had no idea. I felt lost, demolished as if someone has crushed me.

I looked at myself, but there was a bleak shadow. I was afraid that this would overtake me. From the windows of my soul I saw a young innocent girl struggling with a savage beast who invaded her purity. She did not win and he overpowered her with his fierce lust, violent movements which killed her. I looked again at this girl. Could it be me? I shuddered and this shadow was here again. His shadow!

It was dark, but darker in my heart. I remained there and looked around me; all I could see were the skies and the stars above, as if I was already there. I did no longer pertain to this world. I remained there, had no force to move, even though I was not far from home.

SHATTERED WINGS

I looked up at the stars, but no one and nothing could bring back my soul. My body felt trapped, locked in a world which no longer welcome it. My soul departed me to relieve me from the pain, but my fragile body was still here, chilling with the waves of fear which surmounted me after that horrendous experience.

Where was I? Did it happen to me?

When I opened my eyes I found myself lying on the ground, half naked. Suddenly it all came before my eyes, the scenes were conjured up before me one after the other, as if to taunt me again. These scenes were more painful, again I was the innocent girl being violated in the car. Apparently, this is where I left myself and now I longed to die. But I was already dead. Then I saw light in the distance. It was a car.

My heart quivered. He was here again. George has come again and this time he would kill me. It was not him. A man in his sixties was driving the car. He stopped his car and asked me
'Do you need some help?'
'No,' I replied as I did not want him to see me in that shameful state.
He looked at me and almost disbelieving me.
'Are you sure?' he insisted.
I stared at him and for a moment, I thought he was going to do the same like George did. He was insisting as if he understood my situation.
'Where do you want to go?'

Courage then took over me like an overpowering emerging slowly. Perhaps, it was my guardian angel.

'Would you take me to the Police Station?' I asked him.

'Yes, of course.'

I arranged my clothes and went into his car. My body was shivering and I felt lost, stranded as if I had become another person, somebody else. The other one remained in the car struggling to be released from George. Again, I was persecuted by thoughts which invaded my consciousness. I could see him again and again, ravishingly raping me. I saw George with lust in his eyes and he was approaching me, he seized me, kissed me and led me to the ground tearing my clothes. The more I resisted, the more he forced himself.

It was all there before me, as if imprinting its mark on my memory and his breath was forever carved on my skin. I was filled with trepidation. What was next? The car stopped and the man stopped and his lips formed into words. Lost in my thoughts, I had barely noticed that we arrived as I was still reliving that fatal incident.

'Miss, here is the Police Station.'

'Ok, thank you,' I said, while preparing to go out.

This man was different, kind for he asked me again 'Are you sure you want to go alone?'

'Yes, and thank you, thank you for everything.'

I walked inside the police station. The building inside the police station was old and cold. I reached the reception. A large man approached me.

SHATTERED WINGS

'Yes? How can I help you?'
I stared at him blankly, for I could not utter any single word as I felt like choking. He looked at me and then said, 'Wait here,' and he went into the other room. I sat on one of the benches and stared at the wall. The room was chilly with old walls peering at me.

Yet, it felt like being somewhere else in another scene. The police office approached me.
'The inspector is waiting for you in the room,' he said, 'Follow, me.'
I did as he told me and found myself in a large room which was well furnished and more modern than the previous one. I was told to sit down. A few minutes later a young dark woman entered the room. She looked at me and introduced herself.

She was Inspector Hilda. She came closer and gazed at me.
'I know what you've been through.' Her warm eyes and words made me talk and feel comfortable.
I told her everything. It wasn't easy to retell, detail by detail, exactly what happened that night, even if the Inspector was a woman. It still felt shameful to recount that dreadful experience. I felt ashamed and dishonest, as if I had brought the experience on myself; the slightest image of my attacker brought back pain and shame within me.

My lips were dry and I still tasted him inside me and it felt like filth overtaking my system. I felt a wretched soul. The inspector was watching me intently and then I heard her say, 'Can you tell me his name?'

I was taken aback. Then I heard myself saying 'I know him.'

'Good, we can proceed against him. We need to have proof to present to court. First we need to take you to hospital.'

My mind was blank and I stared at her, drowning in the silence of pain.

'Did you say court?' I asked her.

She nodded and her answer threw me into a sea of confusion. Did I have the courage to denounce him? George was a very prominent man, there was no doubt that he would surely get out of this case. Then I recalled his words. No, I could not do it.

The Inspector was awaiting my response.

'What are we going to do Francine?'

'No, it's better if I do not proceed'.

She looked puzzled. 'So you will not proceed?'

'No.' I insisted.

The Inspector moved from her seat and paced around the room.

'Think it over again, but I do not recommend that you stop. Look at yourself, what you had to go through the ordeal. He can do it again to someone else and even to you again. Think about it, but please hurry because we will need the evidence.'

No, I could not do it, I thought. He was stronger than me. I pictured myself in the cold room at hospital, half naked, lying for hours on the couch being examined internally by the doctors whom I knew so well. They would be taking swabs from within me. No, I could not do it. How could I face them without feeling the waves of shame and humiliation overtaking me as they gaze at me again? The scene of the examination will always stand between my duties. Then the scenes of court came before my eyes and I shivered as I visualised myself testifying against him, describing in detail the scene of rape, of him penetrating me as he did it moment after the other. No, this was too much to handle. Also, George was a well known man and I would have to endure the endless attack and questions from the local media. It would be a scandal; it would bring him to shame or to his glory. I could not accept that harsh reality which peered at me cynically from the small window in the room.

'No, I do not want to report,'
I said, more confused than before.

I got up from my seat and walked out of the room away from the Police Station. I didn't have the slightest idea of how to get home, but somehow I managed. This reality was walking with me. Minute by minute I kept seeing the horrid scene. There was only him in my memories and yet, at the same time, I was feeling remote from this world. Yes, as if I belonged to somewhere else.

Silence dominated the whole house and I was determined to keep this silence. No one had to be informed about this experience as if nothing has happened, yet, it happened. I ran up to my room, perplexed and my mind brooding over the recent horrid scene provoked by that recent event. The room was silent waiting for me to return, but there was another me. I took off my clothes filled with dust and filth to remind me of my experience. I headed to the bathroom and prepared to have a shower in a hope it would banish the effects of the rape.

I could still smell the odour of cigarettes and alcohol, the imprints of his breath. . Disgusted, I hoped that the flow of water would cast away his shadow. Fresh water covered my body, but my skin still felt dirty as he, the rapist, was there under my skin. Tears were my only solace that night, like a child longing to go back into her mother's womb.

I no longer belonged there and it was only despair, sadness and misfortune which came unexpectedly all over me. Then I burst into tears of despair and I felt relieved, at least for a while. Water splashed over my body, cleansing the debris from my skin. Not my thoughts, I felt unclean stained with his footsteps.

In my bedroom, the window was slightly open, with rays of the moon softly entering my room. The moon was at its fullest, weaving in her womb, celebrating the Goddess. What Goddess? Mine was burnt in the fire of Hell, like the woman, I have been burnt because of her presumptions they were witches or sorcerers. That was ages ago, but the pain is still the same, permeating my inner labyrinth. The walls of the room suffocated me and I felt like a prisoner locked within my own chains.

SHATTERED WINGS

I looked at my reflection in the mirror and was shocked to see the other woman looking back at me. She was someone else, different from the beautiful Francine. This was another person and her eyes drowned in tears, large and immersed in despair. Was she Francine? No, I felt sorry for her and I wanted to cry with her to make her feel understood.

She smiled at last. Yes, Francine, you need to be strong. Do not be afraid. I am, yet I am not quite sure if the other Francine will ever smile again.

That was the beginning of the two persons living inside me. I had become two persons living a lie. Many days passed and nights where neither the radiant sun nor the glorious moon could reach me. I lived in the dark, buried deep in the underground beneath my soul, as I could not conceal the memories of rape. Perhaps I never will. Part of me longed to forget, cancel the past whilst the other was still in chains and twined to the experience.

Who will win?

But I chose to go on living, hiding underneath this lie which I embedded in deep long silence. Yet, each day brought the pain and the suffering back to me as vivid as if it was actually happening again. I saw it happening every day, as if really was taking place again. The memory relived in my psyche and could not go. It will never go. I returned to work as usual. Days were hard, but I could not reveal what I have been through on that dreaded night. It was not easy, but my life had to go on and the patients could not wait. And this was what gave me hope.

Other days dawned like the previous ones; these were hard, almost unbearable where the memories were crystal clear. Indeed, I was a slave to the memory of rape, a vessel to that night. My heart felt heavy and my life appeared useless, and in these instances the taunting thoughts of suicide were not uncommon, but I never tried.

I thought of my family and my friends who did not know what I went through. They say that death by suicide is not for the departed, but for my loved ones. No, I did not want to leave unanswered questions which will taunt my memory. I did not want to let them know. Yet, doubts persecuted me and came to shatter my peace of mind, as if there was peace before the event. If only I reported him! If I had proceeded against him then things would have taken a different turn, the Inspector's words echoed in my ears. What if he did the same to someone else? My heart ached. Then I would never forgive myself for letting him doing it to other women. Most likely these men do it again.

But what if I reported him? George would have been brought to Justice? He was an important man, with a charismatic flair, and no one would believe he could do this. George was a well known man and he would most probably be protected. That was certain.

SHATTERED WINGS

These thoughts seemed to console me a bit and alleviate the shame and remorse which overwhelmed me, but the deep void within me still lingered like an upbraiding shadow entwined with my soul. I could never forgive him. George was the reason for all of my suffering and I knew that as long as my days were counted there would be no peace.

It is often noted that time can bring hope perhaps even a new life. This was not so in my case. Well, the ordeal had to go on as there was another shocking piece of news waiting to be unfolded. I wasn't feeling well at work, perhaps due to lack of sleep, or lack of food, but these were not uncommon symptoms after a dreadful night which left me lifeless. I kept feeling strange discomfort in my stomach and I knew it was not from lack of food.

While I had been medicating a patient I felt it again and the pain in my stomach came back again, even stronger. My feet dragged me to the bathroom to vomit. I felt sick, but I could not talk about it. This was the result of that dreadful, dark night, a trenchant thought which overpowered me and this amplified my consternation.

This was kept in silence.

Two months passed, but for me they seemed eternity, a never ending affliction. Now, I hoped that death would come and take me. It did not come. This torture persisted and every night I was transported back to that experience. Though I endeavored to bury this experience inside me, my mother seemed to have noticed this. We were in the dining room having dinner, the only time when we could be together. She was watching me intently.

'Francine, are you ok?' she asked.

'Yes,' I lied.

'You look pale and you're not eating.'

'I am on a diet,' I said again.

She looked at me baffled.

'Diet? You don't need a diet.'

I was expecting this reaction from her.

She stared at me, reading my thoughts, and I tried to evade her gaze. Then I continued.

'Of course I do need. I have gained a bit of weight.'

'Francine, I'm your mother, it's not the diet.'

'It is the diet, I have had no time for exercise,' I insisted nervously.

But I knew that my mother was not registering this.

'No, there is something. Francine, we don't even have time to talk to each other like before.'

'It's because I have a lot of work and I feel exhausted after work.'

'You've been working for quite a long time and you never acted this way.'

Her words made me lose my temper. I rose from my chair.

'Mama would you please, leave me alone?' I yelled.

She looked at me seriously, 'Francine, what s' happening to you?'

'I told you, it's the diet.'

SHATTERED WINGS

I walked out of the dining room and rushed to my room; I threw myself on the bed and cried.
Why did I act this way? I didn't blame my mother; she was just caring for me.

Then the pain in my stomach came back as if to confirm my situation. It was unbearable and I had to go to the bathroom to vomit. This seemed to release the pain, but when I went back to my bed scenes kept coming before my eyes. The monster was back and I was dead, killed by the man who raped me and now there was nothing left for me. I saw him again. The brutal monster was penetrating me fiercely and I could not release myself. Again, I felt vulnerable, defeated by lust.
Then Ivan came. He was kissing my lips and uttering sweet words of love. Where was he? Where was I? I had no idea; part of me was wandering alone, disoriented and lost in a labyrinth of end, no return.

Why is Francine still alive? I thought. She could have died. Then Francine would be released from her shadow. With these tormented thoughts I drifted into sleep which could have easily turned into the worst nightmare. I was becoming two people, and I feared I was being deranged by these thoughts. There was a woman deep inside me who remained trapped in that night, to its effect. Another woman struggled to go on, but had no strength.

One afternoon I fainted. This occurred while I was working in the long corridors of the ward.

Suddenly, I felt all the walls surrounding me, my limbs felt weak and I felt myself falling, hitting the ground. I closed my eyes and felt myself being transported to a scene near the sea. Then I heard a man's voice. I was shocked, it was George. No, not again.

'Are you ok?'

Fortunately, it was not George, but Dr Kenneth, one of our young doctors.

Where was I?

His warm eyes brought me back to reality. I saw myself lying on a couch. He spoke again, 'You fainted and your blood pressure is very low.'

I stared at him looking blankly. How did it happen? I could not remember anything. 'You'll be fine, you need some rest.'

Something was happening in my body for which I had no explanation. Perhaps, death was planting its roots deep inside me. I closed my eyes and hoped to rest.

These fainting spells were endless, along with the vomiting and so I decided to go to the doctor. My periods stopped and now my fears were heightened. No it could not be. God forbid. But where was God? God no longer dwelled in my heart. God walked out of my life on that night when George raped me. I felt dirty and could not dare look again at the God who deserted me. He was now far away.

SHATTERED WINGS

The walls in the waiting room were painted white, with pictures hanging on the wall. Nice colours, but no rainbow could console me now. The walls which stared at me were mocking me, my heart was burdened and heavy, for in the coldness of the walls I could sense what was awaiting me. It felt like a spirit warning me. I was in a trap.

After a couple of hours waiting which flew like minutes I was called in. The sympathetic doctor smiled at me. She looked at the file and I could only hope that they promised good news.

Instead, it brought terrible news which pierced me like cold knives.
'Your results are positive for pregnancy,' she started by saying.
Her words struck me like thunder and echoed in my ears like disturbing drums. This could not be.

Then I thought of the brutal persistent way he was thrusting himself inside of me. My heart quivered. I pondered on this sudden reality which descended upon me. It has been my first time and I was not protected. But how could it happen? No, I could not believe this was happening to me. The doctor was watching me intently, but I was only seeing George penetrating me, using his force to instill his seed and impregnate me. He succeeded.
'Is everything ok?' she asked.
'Well, yes,' I lied endeavoring to conceal my embarrassment.

Scenes kept coming before me, like a sequence. He was there forcing and forcing. So he managed to do it and I was most likely in my fertile days. It was made without love, yet I conceived.

No, this was a nightmare. How could it have happened? Perhaps there was a mistake. My mind was thrown into a whirlwind of confusion. The scenes appeared again, flashing in my mind. George was running after me, he had contaminated me with his blood, and now I was carrying him in my veins.   This child was the seed of lust, of violence, of sin and I did not want it. I paid the doctor and hurried out of the clinic.

You're pregnant, pregnant!

The doctor's words kept hammering in my ears. Was it another nightmare? I walked, not knowing where I was heading.

My feet took me to the sea, the sea where I shared my dreams with Ivan and the crystal waves shared my passion and danced with the beatings of my heart. It seemed ages ago, almost like another life time. I stared at the pebbles on the sandy beach, golden reflecting the sun. Not in my heart. All was taken by the wind, and I only wanted to die and ebb away with the waves. I hurried for the beach, feeling the sands contaminating my feet, not unclean like my spirit.   The poor child I was carrying, but I will put an end to it. I walked and walked till I reached the waters.

SHATTERED WINGS

Trumpets were blaring in my ears, noises suffocating me, but it will soon end. The water felt cold, chilly on my skin, it almost burned me. A little pain and it will pass and this hell will be over. Then I thought of the little soul inside me, an innocent child conceived on the night of sin of violence. Images of her diabolical father appeared before me. Then I pictured this undesired child growing up into a beautiful child, her dark eyes staring at me questioningly as she asks.
'Mama, tell me about papa.'

I saw myself bewildered. What would I tell her? That her father raped me? Of course not! I would have to lie to her. I'll tell her that her father was a gentleman, a nice man who died after a terminal illness, or in an accident. She would accept it, it would make her feel good, content, but I would not live that lie. Every time I look in my daughter's eyes I would see him, and again I would smell the fierce odour of his breath, plunging over me and her eyes would remind me of how she was conceived

My God! Who could offer me solace?

George was still there, then the image changed and instead of the child I was seeing him. The water was covering my body and his hands were all over my body again. There was pain as his shadow crept over me. No. I can't carry his child. No. Then a sweeping force took over me and I felt myself being carried away, back to the shore. It was not me, I found myself on the sands and I cried.

Tears were my only company that night, as life has become a train or dark clouds. And it all started by the deception of love. I was cursed, touched by the fierce, menacing claws of evil. What have I done to deserve this? A proper young woman doing her job with love and dedication, was this the reward?

You were a woman. Not your fault, a voice answered deep within me. So, because I was a woman I had to go through all this, there were other women before me and I thought of the women in the books I've read about women in the middle ages, women in war.

Are we the weaker sex or?

I thought of the rape and went back to the scenes and I wondered who was weaker.

Days passed and the secret grew within me, inside my womb. Unwillingly I carried it, uncertain of what step was next. Every dawn brought an agony of doubts and questions. I was certain that I could not keep the child; there were too many memories of that appalling episode in my life. The child was a scar and I could not love it, nor even try. Thinking of it, his seeds growing in my womb repulsed me.

Work for me continued, but I have lost that zest, that love for nursing which so filled my life. There was an over burdening pain which I carried. The first attempt to die did not succeed. Something will come up…I was sure. I did not want the child and fate was surely going to interfere like it did in other days.

I was afraid that it would show…but I was still in the early stages. No one noticed. My father and my friends could not detect anything. Well I made sure that I protect my secret. But I felt rotten. I wonder and marvel at myself, how I kept going on with my life. I had two obstacles to face and they haunted me day and night, the never ending memories of the rape and the child. The future seemed blurred, and all I could see was tunnels leading into darkness, a vacuum…. nothingness.
The breath of life came in my lungs with each dawn, but I was not living, only existing in the form of a number.

Yet, life was still flowing like a silent river.

And there were other days when I did think about the little creature inside me. Poor soul! I felt sorry for my child being introduced to this cold world which already rejects him or her. The child was innocent, but I could give her the love she deserved. I was not the one to give her this love as my heart was dry and there was no warmth in my womb as it was stained with foul of sin. My heart, which once dreamed of pure love, was enclosed within walls of stones which did not let it breath. The circumstances around my child's conception were rather harsh, the result of an unwanted violence. But I felt sorry for it…thought I could not handle it. It was too much for me. For some people, night returns to alleviate them from the heavy burdens of the day, for others it meant holding their beloved in the warmth of their heart. When night returned for me, it brought only darkness, where it took me back to those horrid scenes which were never going to leave me.

At length I gave up the struggle and learned to adjust to them, so much that its effect had become a part of me. I believed that in acceptance, the soul finds its way to peace again. I hoped that one day I would find it. The sheer reality was that I was accepting my experience but not its aftermath.
And that was the child.

Spring in the Mediterranean can be compared to paradise, with the sun warming even the slightest clouds, shining yet, not so strong. The warm rays of the sun felt like warm honey caressing the skin.

It was a promise to the forthcoming season of summer.

It is the best time of the year to linger in the sun, embracing the soft breeze merging with the suns rays the day appear like silk.

That afternoon I was sitting at Café *Cordina*, an open air cafe popular with the inhabitants and even tourists. In the centre a bronze statue of Queen Victoria stands out, reminding us of her glorious days. This is one of the many monuments on the island to remind us of the years governed by different nationalities; the Knights of St. John, the French and the British. But perhaps what makes it

SHATTERED WINGS

distinct from other cafes is the pleasure or privilege of embracing the warm rays of the sun bestowing on the square while drinking a warm coffee or snack.

The sun was caressing my cheeks while I was sitting and having coffee with my friend Sarah.
For one moment, after my experience of rape I was embracing peace. Perhaps the warm rays of the sun helped to caress my heart and to alleviate the pressure. Also, with Sarah I felt at ease and I could talk to her about anything, though I could never share my last experience even though I knew she would have understood.

Today I was feeling good, temporary relieved from the nausea and discomfort which pregnancy brings to its bearers. I smiled broadly, for I could not remember the last time which I could smile from the heart, and while we were chatting, discussing and gossiping my eyes fell on a little angel sitting with his mother on the opposite table. A two-year old boy was looking at me.

I felt a pang in my heart. His big round eyes bored into me and I stared at him. I thought of my child and a shiver ran all over my body. What contrasting reality. I watched the young boy, his round face and big eyes. How I wished he was mine and at that moment the petals of my heart were opened again. Without realising my right hand moved towards my belly. It is there where my boy or girl was resting, waiting to be formed, to be introduced to the world. This was my first contact with my child, it brought tears to my eyes and for the first time I felt the bond between us. A shiver ran all over my spine but then was soon animated by the warmth of the sun.

I smiled at myself, and I felt a new energy rising up in me.

That was a twist in my path which made me change my mind. With this new feeling warming my heart, I decided to keep the child and continue with my pregnancy. Of course, I was aware now of the consequences, but in spite of the fact that this pregnancy was going to be a constant reminder of the rape, I was going to be a good mother.

The days before me were hard, and where I was threading on hard rocks which pierced my feet. Yet, now I wanted it, after staring in the eyes of that angel my feelings took a different turn. His eyes permeating my soul were like those of God. Perhaps there was God after all. But an inner perception feeling still prevailed within me.

I wished that things were different.

If only fate was different…then I would be expecting…Ivan's child, but he betrayed me, lied to me. When I muse about the sequence of events and Ivan's betrayal my heart mellows. Ivan's actions appeared rather mild when compared with George's forced actions. In the warmth of the sun melting the stones in my heart, I could forgive Ivan for deceiving me, but not George. That was utterly impossible. He was out of my life, even though he was everywhere on the media, on papers. It did not bother me, not in the least. People saw in him an honest politician; I saw the other side of him; the beast, the criminal, the rapist who thrived on his lust and sexual perversions to get what he wants. Perhaps this lay hidden in every man. Who knows? It did not annoy me. I hated all men.

But when I thought that he was out of my life, away from my vibrations, he reappeared again. Like a ghost pleading to be heard, but this was no ghost but a fierce monster. Exactly when I had made up my mind to keep the child and to tell my parents about it, to face all the hurdles and situations faced by single mothers, George appeared again, to haunt me, to torment me, to destroy my life and destruct the seeds within me. His seeds became violent again, like him. Looking back, I regret it for the price I paid was far too high.

For some unknown reason, fate had made an oath to disrupt every step I took and now that I had made up my mind up to keep my child, George called me again at my place of work. I was astounded to hear his voice again.
'What do you want of me?' I asked him firmly.
He answered with his charming calm tone of a politician ready to impress.
'I want one last thing,' he said.
Hadn't he had enough? I felt an urge to tell him everything, but something held me back. I could not, he was an outsider. Yes, an outsider who invaded me.
'George, leave me, I am busy.'

He replied.

'I know that, but to remind you not to speak about what happened that night.'

I remained speechless, staring blankly at the ceiling. George was still thinking of what happened that night. Was he regretting it, feeling the heaviness of guilt overpowering him? I doubted it. The men who rape and violate women have no feelings. Then it dawned upon me. The elections were coming up and he was protecting his name. What a callous man! Only his reputation mattered.

He spoke again.

'Francine, it was all your fault, don't you dare speak or you'll be in deep shit.'

I cut the line and my hands were shaking. How could he do that to me?

My heart was breaking into pieces and a chill ran all over my body. When was I going to break these chains? What a fool I had been to think that George was out of my life, out of my path. Yet, he was still present, menacing me like a consistent dark shadow, stalking me. He did it once and he seemed adamant in his goals to shut my mouth to safe regard his position and I let myself be buried in endless silence. I did not report him and proceed against him but buried his sin within me.

Why? Well, it was the obvious truth. George was a politician, an important person on the island. He could not afford to be hindered by his deeds. Like every politician he had to keep appearance, appear untouched, virgin, and indulged with virtue.

SHATTERED WINGS

But I knew his sin.

I hurried away from the desk and went to my work feeling perturbed by his phone call. This played a part in the next twist of fate. My heart was suddenly closed again, protected by huge walls which surmounted it. That was the best way. Suddenly, even the creature within me had become him, my enemy. I loathed George, wished him all the sufferings, all the unhappiness on this earth. I wished him death. The creature inside of me was constantly reflecting his shadow, the monster that raped me and took away my happiness. George had to be eliminated too, perhaps then that night would be banished forever from my memory.

I had to put an end to all this, once and for all. How dare he call again? Almost after three months of torments, of engulfing the secret deep inside of me, again he tried to use his power to threaten me. Perhaps, this was another form of power.

I had to go on with my life. I longed to go back to that innocent girl who once walked in the corridors, opening her heart to her patients. Then she opened her heart to men and she stumbled in her path. They burned the flower residing inside her and now she was stained, almost drowned and perished with the wind of devastation. I thought of the day when I tried but did not succeed. The same feelings were coming again and I hated him and could not even forgive him. He destructed my life. And there was no turning back.

I was ruined forever, blemished with the evil of his soul. Not only did he abuse me, but he left his mark in my womb which now has become tarnish like him. I detested him and deplored the thing which I carried inside me. It was a thing, for me no pure soul or pure life could be conceived by that monster.

The sooner I got rid of it the better. There were many women who had it before me and will keep on doing it. That was what I was going to do. An inner urge propelled me to get rid of it, for the more I thought of it the more I felt myself abominating this little thing or creature being formed inside of me.

The pain, the nausea was a constant reminder of George and his malicious act. There were no regrets inside of me, for I could not go on nurturing the devilish seeds weaved in Hell. Who could blame me? Now nothing could change my mind, I was determined to get rid of it, the heavy burden which was my curse would haunt me for the rest of my days. I could not even think of adoption. No, the thought of having a living child somewhere would haunt me for eternity; I would never ever grow to love it. Abortion was the cure. At least it was the solution for that moment, but I needed to do something as I longed to be free.

Being a Catholic country, Malta considers abortion as illegal.

It is against God, a crime against life, but when a woman is raped, forced to do unwanted sexual acts, abortion becomes the sole relief. Children may be considered a gift from God, but only when conceived out of love…. I presume.

Of course, being a nurse, I exerted myself to save lives and this was rather in contrast with my principles, where on principle I was against killing, above all, an innocent child. Being in the actual situation is different. This was not irresponsible sex without protection based on the presumptions of intense pleasure and gratification. This was the result of a monstrous act of forced violence. I was even a virgin when I was raped and now I have to carry this burden by myself. Not only did I have the misfortune of getting pregnant, but also being raped by a powerful man.

I was overpowered by his violence and by his position. I could not go on with this pain any longer, or else I would have to die. At the same time the courage to do it, to douse the flames of my fire had deserted me. Perhaps I was not living any longer. Quite possibly I died on that night when Francine was raped. Yes, my soul was taken with the stars. If only I could shut my eyes forever, then this would be over. It would stop here.

I know that moralists may preach that life starts upon conception, and that it's not right to kill. It is murder in their eyes and before God…, but are men allowed to rape? Rape! The word sends shiver all over me and my soul feels enchained in a deserted unknown abyss. The reality is that a woman cannot bear to be reminded of the violence imposed on her.

For me, rape is actually a mild form of murder. Yes, murder of the spirit. No, I was certain now. There were moments when I tried to envisage myself rearing the child after birth, but this was utterly impossible. He would be there to remind me of how he was introduced in the world, by the seeds of violence. I pictured him looking at me like that child did under the warm spells of the sun. Instead I saw hatred and power in his eyes. I saw George looking through the windows of his son's eyes. I shuddered, as I thought of Juan, the light in his eyes. He was gone now. But my child did not have this light in his eyes. I would grow to hate him and that would be another sin, the seeds of hatred. They were already there, planted deep within my heart which replaced every dream of love which I could have had.

And that was beyond me.

I wanted to break free and after releasing this thing I would go abroad, then I would be free from the past. So my mind was set and I formulated my plans. At least my life was moving. A window was opened for me and I tried to look at the view, hoping I would grow to love it. At least there was that hope in my heart. During my hours at work, I managed to do some research on where to end my pregnancy. Someone told me that there was a doctor in the Northern part of Malta who could help me, I felt relieved. A few more days and I would be born again.

There were moments during those days when I wished I could go back, but the voyage to freedom had commenced and I could not go back. Even if I wanted to, there was no turning back. Still, residing in my memory there was the picture of that boy with angelic eyes peering at me. He was haunting me and I could still see him looking at me, smiling. He could be the child in me, but no, my child would be a devil. No hard feelings, he had to go, and so must George, out of my mind, out of my life.

The doctor was very helpful. He explained to me the procedure and nothing was new to me. I knew it was hard for both of us and for my future to go through the endless memory of having aborted a child, but then I was carrying within me remnants of a terrible night. I was offered no choice. It was too late when I learned about the consequences which rape had sown weaved inside me.

That night I had a dream, I saw myself standing over the edge of a cliff. Strangely, though in the dream it was me, I was much younger, a little girl. Then, the teddy bear which I was holding slipped from my hands and fell down, deep into the cliffs. I woke up startled. My hands were clammy and my body sweating. What was I doing? It was only a dream, I reassured myself. Yet, it could also mean that I was being freed from my burden, and this brought me relief.

The day dawned and I was going to spend the week end away. I told my mother that I was on a week end in Gozo with my friends. I could not face her; I lacked the courage to look into her eyes. Mine were full of lies, concealing a sequence of events. I could not share my secret with anyone and no one would know what I kept inside my soul.

I've cried enough, but what appeared most was the mask which I wore every day, and beneath that mask there was a dead woman, hiding behind the veil of suffering. I was not sure if it was really me hiding under that veil.

I walked into the place alone. A couple of hours more and my Hell would vanish, ebb away with the wind.

The last minutes were Hell, as if they were there to taunt me and perhaps make me go back on my decision. I kept coming across children and women expecting children. Was this a test to make me change my mind and turn direction? At the same time I envied the woman who had the courage I lacked.

Suddenly my feet faltered and my heart pondered.

A shiver ran all over my body, the women were loved by their men, while I wasn't. Their children were conceived out of love in the warmth of passion and desire. Mine was conceived in utter darkness, ravishing my innocence which I held for the man who would love me one day. There was no one, and even when I tried to open my heart to them it was rejected. I was savagely abused, left alone, left with no choice and perhaps killing George's seed was driven by an unconscious desire driven by revenge.

That was what distinguished us. I felt a twinge of pain and now I hated the children walking about, I resented the women, and their bellies seemed to be mocking me. Soon mine would fade. Soon I would be a new woman, and this gave me the courage to keep on walking on the path which I firmly believed in. Whereas, I thought I would be indifferent to this act, having no feelings or remorse, but the reality was otherwise.

While I sat on the bed, many thoughts crossed my mind. Never had I felt so close to the child inside me, not even on that day when I decided to keep it. No, the child was hammering inside me, urging me to let it stay there in the warmth of my womb, but my womb was cold and dry and could not welcome it. The child inside of me wanted to live and was defying me and struggling to go on. What was I doing? What this a parallel reality?

I pictured myself in the delivery room, waiting for my child to be born, forcing my movements to bring forth a new life, a normal delivery where the woman introduced her baby to this world, but what sort of world awaited my child? It was a cold lonely, world constructed on walls of abuse, and giving my child away to the Angel of Death was protecting it from this world. This seemed to soothe me and focus on my goal.

I closed my eyes and thought of the Angel of Death. Today he was stroking my cheek, fondling my hair. I would rather be touched by him then by rage of violence and sexual aggression.

Rape is the Angel of Death, so my child had already been introduced to death on the day it was conceived.

No, I did not want my child to recall the forceful movements of his father's body thrusting inside me, and the pain, the humiliation which I had to carry for the rest of my life. Every time I look into my child's eyes, George's eyes would be there, penetrating mine, invading me. No. This had to stop. Then I felt stronger.

In a private room, I lay on a couch, naked from the waist down and my legs wide open. A shiver ran all over my body. It was chilly. I closed my eyes and thought of George, when he spread my legs open and forced himself on me. Now he was there, reincarnated and forced inside my belly. My womb rejected him, like I had been once. It could no longer dwell there.

I thanked myself for taking the decision.

Other women would condemn me for this immoral act, but after rape one is devastatingly oppressed and has no control on life, and pregnancy becomes an extra strain. At the same time I knew it would have side effects, physical, emotional, psychological, but I wanted to go on with it. The thought of George made me do it; I detested his blood teeming deep inside of me. The emotions which came overwhelmed and confused me. Part of me wanted to let go, the other wanted to keep the child. An inner voice admonished me; you did not succeed in taking your life and now you are taking someone else.

The child was the spawn of a monster. Then, all of a sudden I felt a quivering movement inside me. It came from my belly, my child was moving, but I could not turn back. A strange feeling took over me. It was this sudden movement which tormented me, but I could not change my mind. This was George's last struggle to keep his domain. No, I could not turn back.

I saw the nurse approaching my side. She took my hands and was preparing to give me an injection. The lights in the room were dim and my eyes flickered and I felt myself being transported into a fog. I saw myself walking in the woods, but my body felt light, my limbs felt like flying, like a free bird. Someone was calling my name, I looked around me and there was no one in the fog. I heard them calling my name and part of me wanted to return, the other part struggled to remain lost in the fog. It was warm and comfortable, freeing me from the heavy burdens of what I had to go through.

Perhaps the dawn of guilt was descending slowly on me. Then I opened my eyes and found myself lying on the couch. I recalled the dream and I longed to remain there away from the reality which surmounted me.

And I felt trapped again.

The dim light was hurting my eyes and it was very cold, my limbs were freezing but so was heart. It was over, and then when I looked around me, I only saw the haziness of the room. There was a strange feeling inside me, I felt knocked out. They left me in the room for some time. Then I was allowed to leave.

It was over, and through the depths of death I longed to be reborn again, to be a free woman, flying like the bird in the dream. I hoped now to meet the other woman whom I left behind in the scene.

Will I ever find her? Will she come again?

There were more paths which I had to walk before encountering this woman again, for she was buried in the immensity of the desert. A feeling of relief swept all over me, and for brief moments I felt happy, or perhaps I made myself believe that I was happy, for deep within me I was not. I knew that I could never be. Yet, I still hoped….

A new person was emerging. Was it? Before the operation, I had been aware that there would be psychological ailments, mood swings to follow me wherever I went. Yet when I was faced with the aftermath of my action, I was faced with a different reality.

A few days later I got consistent cramps and I even bled. These physical ailments took me back in time, where my body recalled the other pain incited by the devil who deflowered me. I never thought it would hurt that much, but this was only a surgical intervention, the other was Hell. Still there were its effects plodding on my soul.

The only reassurance was that it would pass. It did not, for these effects were to persist, as if to remind me constantly of my sin. It suddenly occurred to me that there was no end to this saga of episodes which plagued me. This was an open wound which could never heal. Every day in my body I felt that sense of emptiness, as if something has been sucked out of me, from deep within me. It felt like my soul had deserted me again and the night has come to haunt me. Indeed, my child, my flesh and blood was taken and dragged out of my womb, which have continued to welcome it. And I put out, ruthlessly, to relieve the pressures on me, hoping to get away from the memory of rape.

The memory of that night was deeply buried within me and the memory of the child was embedded, clinging to every cell inside my body, perhaps to instill within me a sense of remorse, or to avenge me for what I have done. These were the feelings which accompanied me. And I realised that I was still not free.

The days were passing rapidly and the sun came up every day with every dawn, but not for me. My life went on, and so did my work, but there was an inner feeling which afflicted me. It was a sense of helplessness, weakness which overruled my days. Though I felt dead I did not surrender and continued with the quest to survive, to overcome the shadow of violence and co come out of my past.

There were moods. For most of the times I felt like crying and felt like being thrown in a river of despair. It was what was left. When I expected the dawn of relief to reach me, it did not and it was only waves of sadness which formed part of my breath. A feeling of emptiness pertained deep within me and my soul was transported in an endless vacuum.

Where was I? Perhaps, I was lost in the fog of the past. Certainly there was something missing, a part of me was left in another part. At the same time I could not determine what was really lacking. Was it part of me, my soul or the child? I could not tell, but I was thrown into a whirlwind of confusion, and I was lost, I felt myself entering in another world, a strange world which was quite unfamiliar.

At least I was free from the memory of rape which constantly haunted me. I thought that this would pass, that I would recover and overlook this experience. It did not. While nights were supposed to relieve me and take me to a journey away from my pains and the experiences, it made things worse for me. Instead, nights came to haunt me and in their stillness they reminded me of my sin, removing life from my womb where it could have thrived. These were the thoughts which haunted me and in the dark, soundless night these inner voices sounded like never ending drums in my ears. The voices sang in chorus, murderer, murderer. And that pierced my heart like daggers, for I was not an assassin, rather the contrary, where I worked hard to save lives. Yet, I did not save my child.

Yes, perhaps I have killed my own child, but I was murdered before I could even express the desire of exerting my maternal instincts. Strangely, it decided for me. In the bitter silence of deep lust, in the heat of utter passion, my life had been mutated by a monster whose aim is only to kill in deep silence when no one can hear the cries of his chosen prey. And in the deepest silence I have killed my child. Now the child has come to avenge me.

These thoughts were suffocating me, choking me, as if I was the one to blame. No, I was not to blame. The child was the seed of sin; the son or daughter of a rapist. Who would want to live knowing that? I comforted myself.

Looking back now at my situation, it suddenly occurred to me that given those circumstances I would not have made it, and the only possible way was to take that decision. Carrying and rearing his child meant the onset of my tribulation.

George was up there, high on a pedestal and if his devious acts were to be revealed to his voters they would without doubt abominate him and he would fall. Yet, he did not, for I did not act. Perhaps, my sole revenge, or triumph lies in demolishing every trace of his evidence inside me, and that was his son. My heart quivers when I think of his other son, the innocent boy who was swallowed by the claws of death. What similarity between but the sheer truth is that George did not deserve their love and their presence in his world.

It was through this devastating truth that I found solace, for this was the only shield left to protect me. He or she could not return back, and this poignant feeling will fade for ever, but then even love was not coming back, was far more to painful.

This grievous thought was to remain with me, creating feelings deep within me of being useless, wretched and dead inside. There was no light, for my life has been utterly demolished and ravished by men.

The days flew by, as they always do, but they did so with no meaning for me. Dawn came only to remind me that I was still breathing, but there was that other part of me who was still struggling. Every day brought with it the deep feeling of loss, making me a slave to myself. I had become a slave again, and this time to myself. Without doubt I have become a slave, but above all, my own worst enemy to my emotions.

Two personalities dwelled within me, and I felt like living in two persons, and none of them belonged to me. Now, days turned into weeks and into months. Determined to leave the past behind me I endeavoured and struggled to keep going and even the effects imposed by surgical abortion were waning, or rather the shadows of that were dissolving into the fog of my memories.
There was nothing that I could do, but certainly I could not go back, and even if the road before me was blurred, my feet had to keep on threading.

It was a strange, unknown path which unfolded before me and I followed its direction.

A new chapter was awaiting me.

The sun with its rays is always a promise to a better life and the radiant soul of summer was preparing to enter our world again, as it did in previous years. It is there that life seems to take a new turn and what seems dull and bleak takes a different light. The summer returned again, promising the same warmth blazing in one's heart. I could feel the rays of the sun on my cheeks and I assured myself that I would seek ways in order to brighten my heart. Perhaps the moon was smiling at my fate, or was rising in my constellation.

Whatever it was, I started to feel better at least for a while. Yet, that terrible night will never leave me, and every fraction of it will remain etched in my memories as long as I live. I can only hope that there will be other dawns which will not be steeped in my recollections of that dreadful day. Meanwhile, I was determined to go forward, and there was a dawn of hope which cascaded on my fate.

One fine day, the first rays of the warm sun opened my breath and instilled inside me the dawn of a new hope, and that was when I met Gino.

I loved the Neolithic Temples, with their golden stones, which once they could have been embodied with lapis. Who can tell? But I knew, and it seemed that these mystical stones were in complete synchrony with my soul. They were the ones which brought me this new light, for in their mystery they had the capacity to take me away from myself and my pains. I felt like a young girl again, marvelling at their greatness. But it did not remain the same. At least looking at them reminded me of the unique and sacred relationship that I shared with them and took me from where I was back to my origins. My heart was feeling heavy, but standing before them helped to cure my heartache. These Neolithic giants stood many years before me, watching over the sea, guiding time and space…watching over my fate!

And that was the same fate which raped me and robbed me from my love. Still I longed to breathe the fresh air, uncontaminated by impure thoughts and bad memories. I longed to feel the spirit of bliss in my lungs again. The temples offered me the promise that day, of somewhere in which I hoped that my soul would be free and flowing with boundless river.

It could all be different now.

One afternoon I finished work early and decided to go out. It was a beautiful day, with the welcoming warmth of the sun. Then it occurred to me that summer was close to us and I thought of the Temples and how every cycle of seasons had an impact on them. All I knew was that I wanted to go there to be with them. Perhaps, there in their stillness I would rediscover the peace that was taken away from me by fate.

My adorable temples remained the same, still standing. I felt them watching intently with their eyes peering at me and filling my soul as if comprehending what I had to go through since the day I left them. I was a little girl then.

That moment I envied them, for they remained intact, pure, representing space and time and the secret knowledge of other planes of reality. I could not see it, but I stood there motionless, just watching them embracing the rays of the sun until it was time to set. I witnessed a magnificent scene, with the red lights on the magnificent stone. I took a deep breath and let myself go with the beauty before my eyes. For the first time, after all the passing events, I felt a warm wave of contentment running all over my body.

Then, to my complete surprise, it occurred to me that I was no longer alone. There was someone in the place. There was someone, who like me relished in the beauty of the temples. Now he came closer, and I saw a shadow cast on the huge stones. The shadow was approaching me and I looked back, startled, but he turned out to be a handsome young man. He was tall, well built and was looking at me. I was taken aback. What did he want?

It was the first time I was alone in the presence of a man since the rape. A feeling of panic took over me but I tried to control myself.

'Hi,' I heard him say. 'It is really nice here.'

'Yes,' I uttered.

Then he introduced himself.

'I am Gino, nice to meet you.'

'Francine,' I said in a low voice and we both shook hands.

'Can I sit beside you?' he asked me.

'Ok,'

He sat on a small rock close to me and started to talk. Mainly, he talked about himself. This was perhaps to start the conversation, but I was feeling uneasy. All I was registering in my mind was the fact that I was alone with a man. All of a sudden I thought of George and felt myself traveling in the past; after all that I had to go through and now I was sitting beside a man. What if he did the same to me?

SHATTERED WINGS

An inner feeling inside me propelled me to run away from my beloved monuments, which were now threatened by a man who represented hatred and violence inherent in all men. The urge was to escape, but there was a strange feeling which compelled me to remain there. There was a part of me which wanted to out flush out the past. So, I stayed there, and my only shelter from any harm was my beloved majestic temples. They watched over time and now they were watching over me. I listened to him while he talked about his life.

Gino was an artist, and he liked to come here and look at the view. At least he sounded different from the other man. His voice was tender, but still I could not trust him. Even though I was happy in his company I was still feeling qualms deep within me.

The feeling that from one minute after the other he could do something like the George was constantly there. It came to haunt me or to warn me that no man could be trusted, no matter how gentle he appeared.

Gino was looking at me and in the warm sunset rays his eyes looked warm, pleading me to trust them. But I could not trust, not even the kindest look could melt my heart. I concluded that behind the gentle look there was a burning fire of violence waiting to be kindled.

It was getting dark and I decided to go. Gino offered to escort me home, but I could not accept.

Never take the risk again, I warned myself. This was a lesson which I learned at a price.

So I walked away from the temples, my mind overcrowded by thoughts and ambivalent emotions. There was no denying that the experience of rape had shaped me into another woman. This woman, who was emerging ploddingly from within me, was incapacitated by fear every time she gets close to a man. That was me, my reality.

Every man conveyed to me the memory of that vile night; they hauled me to the nightmare which persecuted me day and night. The shadow of violence had turned me into a fierce creature, even to the extent of murdering my own child. If only he hadn't come to remind me of my vulnerability, of the hidden memories of utter darkness! I longed to embrace the beauty of the temples, to let myself go with the waves of time. Yet, I could not do it. Now, there was this shadow haunting me. But I yearned to be loved by a man, to love them back and share the passion and affection. I knew that this was a remote dream which could never be fulfilled. Possibly this type of man did not exist on this planet. Who knows? I thought about how far can men change their skins and descend into shadows of violence sends chills all over my body. I could never trust a man.

And this thought enslaved me.

My journey away from the experience of rape was a long one, and set in motion in my life an endless crusade against legions of thoughts, moods and mixed emotions, of which I was often their own creator. Days were vague and no day was like the other. There were days which only dawned to revive the memories again, where the events surfaced again. They were clear and vivid as if they were reoccurring again. Other days came where these events seem to melt into nothingness, ebb away into air.

This has become a cycle which carried me away with the waves, yet the wheel of my life kept rotating with my life, or else my existence. Lessons in life are continuous and my life was no exception. Perhaps this lesson was needed for my healing? And Gino was part of this lesson.

*

The streets of Valletta were overcrowded with people rushing to shops or back to their offices. By contrast, I was walking placidly, without letting any thoughts afflict me, for I longed to be free with every slow step that I made. Nevertheless, I did succeed.

The next step which I took was not a ponderous one like the ones before it. As I walked along, unaware, I thought I heard someone calling my name. It was a man's voice, and all of a sudden all my serenity vanished.

I thought of that malicious voice of the evil man who destroyed my days. I turned away and kept walking hastily yet, the voice persisted. Then it occurred to me that this was not the menacing sound of that monster. Then who was it? I thought, but the warm voice calling my name was familiar.

He was Gino, the man at the temples.
'Francine,' I heard him say.

His voice took me back to that majestic scene of the sun setting over the temples and the interesting conversation I had with him. He was here now. I turned around and there he stood, watching me intently. I stared at him and in broad daylight he appeared more handsome. He had black curly hair tinted with grey and pale skin which made him look attractive. I guessed Gino must have been in his early forties, but what struck me were his eyes which were small and dark but warm.
'Hi,' I said.
'Do you remember me? We met at the temples.'
Of course I remembered him. How could I forget the scene at the temples? 'Yes, yes.' I replied.
'And you are Francine! Am I right?'
So he remembered my name. I looked at him bewildered.
'Yes.'
'I never forget a beautiful woman.'
'Thanks,' I said, at a loss for words.
Gino must have sensed this for he said, 'I ordered a book and came to collect it..... And you?'
'No, I also came to buy something.' I heard myself saying.
'Good! Francine would you like to join me for a coffee?" he asked me.

SHATTERED WINGS

I hesitated. Should I go? The warmth in his eyes allayed my fear and so I joined him for coffee. We walked for some minutes and then went in a nearby cafe. I must admit that I was enjoying the company of Gino quite delightful. He came into my life in those days when the memories started to wane, just for a while.

Gino taught art at university, but was also an accomplished artist. Artists are supposed to be free spirits who view life in its full form. They have the ability to go within all levels of life. But Gino was a man. The overshadowing doubts had become my solace and my only warning.

In spite of all these thoughts and fears which tormented me, there was a part within me that wanted to love again. A new wave of excitement swept all over me. Perhaps my life was going to take a different path at last, or the energy and affectionate attention of Gino was beaming new light in my life. This man was trying to mend my broken pieces, shattered as I was by life.

Something strange was happening, and without realising I, was feeling being drawn to this man. Was this the first sign of love? If this was the case, then it was surely good news which brought relief to me. Yet, even if the first wing beats of love were brushing against my heart, it could not be the same passion, the same beatings of my heart for Ivan. No, that was buried in the desert which will never return.

What I felt for Gino was a special affection and a sense of pleasure in his company and after what I had been through, this feeling presented the first onset of healing. Possibly, it was the other woman who was attempting to play this part of flirting, loving and moving away from the pain and humiliation she had to endure. The other woman was left buried with only the stars to recount her story.

Again, I did not know which part was leading my life.

Gino promised me to show me his studio, so one evening I joined him to see his art works. It was comprised of large rooms with works all over them. It was exhilarating to see his paintings and as I walked round I had to stop and contemplate at the beautiful portraits, sculptures and paintings of nudes and temples.

The beauty of art rendered me breathless, and admiring the works one after the other I felt myself being overwhelmed by this magical world of art. The world shared by the man whom I was beginning to like, just when I thought that my life was over. Gino walked with me and remained silent looking at his works. All of the paintings were appealingly beautiful, but I could not help but admire the paintings depicting the temples. They were eloquent and enchanting. I felt enraptured where the temples penetrated my soul and endeavored to revive the light inside it.

SHATTERED WINGS

Gino was watching me intently then he broke the silence,' What do you think?'
'Beautiful,' I uttered.
'I am glad you like my paintings.'
'A lot,' I responded.
His lips formed into a smile revealing his lines around the corner of his eyes.
'I got my inspiration from the temples.' he added.
'Really?' I asked him.

Indeed. The temples are a source of inspiration for everyone. Gino gripped my hands and looked deeply into my eyes.
'Francine, I must tell you something.'
He paused but his eyes were fixed on mine.
'That evening was special for me. It's because I met you.'
I liked his words, but then he was coming closer and closer and his lips were becoming closer now. A shiver ran all over my spine and I felt a lump in my throat. He was going to kiss me, but I could not let him. I liked him and my lips yearned to taste the sweetness of love, to open my heart again and to let myself drown into the sea of passion. I had never been there and the only time was under the devastating shadows of violence. Now, my body and my heart longed to go there.

Yet, no...

No, Gino was kissing me on my lips, sweet promise of love and passion, but my mind was whirling. Tormenting thoughts of Ivan came before my eyes. I thought of him and recalled his touch and his kisses which then vanished, gone with the wind for he deceived me. Then the appalling images of George appeared and that aggravated the situation.

Was Gino the same?

Even though I liked him and longed to return his kisses, there was something inside me which held me back. An inner force compelled me and I moved back.
'No Gino.' I said firmly.
Like a gentleman, that he was, Gino stepped back. Then he said, 'I am sorry. I rushed.'

Gino caressed my hair and kissed me on my cheeks and at that moment I could not but admire him. It grieved me though, that I was not free to express what I really felt for this man. Perhaps, one day I would, but that day might not dawn at all.

We then kept walking around the room, and the amazing paintings were witnessing the scene between us. It made me feel a failure and vulnerable again, but the works of art were consoling me, the colours healing my wounds. Then a lovely painting of a nude caught my attention. The woman was lying in a reclining position, her flesh her contours well defined. Gino was surely a great artist.

'Tell me about this nude,' I remarked, also to divert myself from the inner torments provoked by the rejection of his genuine advances. He walked closer to the picture.

'Yes, I painted her three years ago, with oils.'

As he talked, his eyes glowed like stars and I listened to him in silence. There was no doubt that I liked this man, the artist who was showing me warmth. The petals of my heart were closed and surrounded by his paintings; I envied them, for they could give him what I could not give him, but I was not going to give up.

That night sleep eluded me and I laid awake, thinking and pondering about my experience. The images kept coming back, I pictured Gino around his paintings, trying to kiss me, to love me and I had rejected him. My heart was frozen, chilled by the harmful events of the past, which suffocated me.

I felt locked in a prison, chained by my thoughts. The warm gaze of Gino kept haunting me, but we were two islands apart from each other. The hours dragged by and I tried to sleep, but it was to no avail. Tossing and turning in my bed, I kept thinking. I visualised myself with Gino, where I was kissing him. Then I shuddered, instead Gino became George and the dream stopped abruptly.

The light of the moon was peering from my window, but I kept seeing the scenes one after the other. George appeared again, walking closer to me, and then he forced himself on me again. I suddenly felt a sharp pain in my pelvis as if I was there again, lying on the ground, as he penetrated me fiercely. I was there again and the emotions flooded all over me, the devastating memories have never left me but were concealed, hiding expecting for the right moment to emerge.

Tears were the only solace.

It was only in the early hours that I managed to get some sleep. When will this come to an end? Just when I thought that I had started the journey away from rape....

Yet, I went on with my life and my work. These tormenting thoughts and memories were buried inside me, but I could not surrender. This struggle had to be fought and won.

Gino was still present in my life. He opened up new avenues for me and he introduced me to the world of art. I accompanied him to exhibitions, lectures and anything which had to do with art. These colourful paintings gave me a new delight, a new life. Gino was a new light. He was calm, warm and understanding, but I could not open myself completely to him.

It was utterly hard to expose myself again, even though I was dying to be loved. It was no use no use denying the fact that Gino loved me, and he made it clear, but I tried to control myself and hide my feelings. Of course I loved him, and wanted to give him all my heart, but I could only dream and even dreams were an ominous reminder of the past.

SHATTERED WINGS

Then it happened again and this was the first step to break the barriers between us. Or at least I hoped so.

One afternoon I joined Gino in his studio where he was working on one of his paintings.
'Hi, come in,' he said.
'Come and see it, it's nearly finished.'

I walked in, went up to him and kissed him on his cheeks. Gino was working on an exquisite painting of a nude young woman. In the painting she was depicted lying on the bed. The model was extremely beautiful, with her flesh being eloquently painted and revealing her contours in detail.

Beautiful and exuberant, the opposite to how I was feeling. A shiver ran all over my body, for the woman in the painting reminded me of myself before the experience. The woman presented purity and intact sensuality, waiting to be touched by the ripples of love. This was all taken from me and the woman inside me had been killed, buried deep in the labyrinths of my unconscious.

Gino was watching me intently, expecting my reaction.
'What do you think, my dear?' he asked me.
'It's extraordinary,' I replied, trying hard to conceal my inner thoughts.
He smiled.
'I am glad you like it.'
He kissed me on the cheeks.

'Who is the model?' I asked curiously.
'She's a model from Bulgaria.'
'She's beautiful,' I retorted.
'Yeah, but beauty goes beyond that.'

I looked at the painting again, but looking at her naked flesh instigated deep within me a twinge of envy. In her pose she expressed a careless freedom about herself and about her body. This model was all that I longed to be and could not be, for I dared not to even look at my body in the mirror. It meant only shame and generated contempt for myself and my body, which was stinging with violence and the dirt of lust.

Gino was saying something.
'Francine,' he said, 'I'd love to paint you someday.'
I stared at him, bewildered. Painting me! Not even in my wildest dreams. I could not compare myself with the woman in the painting! How could I reveal myself again....even though a part of me desired to be painted by him?

Deep down I knew that this could not be. I was ruined and did not even belong to my body, even to myself. Gino was waiting for my response. He put his hands around my shoulders.
'Tell me you accept.'
'I don't know,' I said perplexed.
'We will see,' he said tenderly.
Then he moved closer and started to fondle my hair.
'Francine, I like you a lot.'

SHATTERED WINGS

Then he moved his hands across my cheeks and started caressing them softly. A shiver ran all over my body and a strange feeling overwhelmed me. I knew the feeling. It took me back to the first touch given by my first love, Ivan. I had feelings for this man, who was warm and gentle. But, he could turn into a monster instantly, in a second. I warned myself, but today I wanted to let myself drown in the sea of his love, to break from the chains which enslaved me. His warm lips were heading for mine and I responded to his kisses. His body was closer to me now and his warmth swept all over my body, creating a wave of bliss. It felt good, like warm waters spreading all over my body and I wanted to go on. This sudden wave of passion brought a sense of relief. For the first time, after months of Hell, I was grasping the gates of ecstasy and I owed it to this man. My limbs felt like shaking with the sudden warmth pouring all over them.

It had been a long time since I experienced that sensation, which I thought was diminished forever from my life. Today, this feeling came back unexpectedly and I wanted to cherish it.

Gino was kissing me ardently and I kissed him back, losing myself in his kisses. It was a lovely feeling taking me away from myself. Then, Gino moved to my breasts, and his hands felt soft, leading me to a dream, which I embraced heartily. His kisses went on taking me away from myself and where the waves of the sea engulfed me in passion which I relished, at the same time cutting the ties of the past.

The lips which were kissing me were forming into words. I followed him and we went upstairs. Gino led me to a large room which was also full of paintings. In one of the corners there was a large sofa and then we lay down on it. Gino started kissing me ardently again, arousing the waves of passions deep within me. I closed my eyes and let myself embark in this new world of ecstasy, freeing myself from all the oppression which submerged me. A new woman was emerging. In the storm of our passion I heard him say, 'I love you, Francine.'

A feeling of elation took over me. His words took me to heaven, but did I love him? Well, yes...

What followed struck me like thunder. The dream had to come to an end. Now, Gino was moving closer and closer, almost thrusting himself inside me. I was going to do it. It had to be the next twist.

In the heat of passion, in his sweet movements of his kisses I prepared to part my legs as part of an uncontrollable attempt, driven by my instincts to welcome him, but I did not succeed. There was intense pain which flooded between my thighs. No, I could not do it. Suddenly Gino became an invader, hurting me and instead of love it felt like a hot poker piercing me. Swiftly I found myself entering into a dark tunnel and all the memories of that night returned again.

I was taken aback again and I found myself in his car and he was hurting me…… and hurting me. The waves of passion which caressed me turned into darkness. This quivering reality had an effect all over my body. My muscles became suddenly tight and cold, and instead of Gino I was seeing George lying on my body, once again. All the scenes came before me. George was trying to penetrate me, to infiltrate his essence.

Now, Gino's lips felt repulsive, and his breath reminded me of that dreaded night.
I could not continue.
'No, no,' I told him.
Gino looked at me, confounded.
'Francine, what's wrong?' he asked me tenderly.
'Nothing… it's that I can't,' I said.

Gino did not utter any single word, but he watched me intently, trying to work out what had happened to me. I knew the reason, but I could not disclose my pain, even though Gino would have understood.

Not yet.…

I knew that my reaction baffled Gino and I could expect any response imaginable. I was ready to accept the consequences. A profound silence reigned between us and in this silence Gino was awaiting my answer. He did not get it.

Instead he reached to kiss me, but I turned my back to hide the tears which were rolling on my cheeks.
'Ok,' he said and then walked out of the room.
Just when I thought it was over, it came back to torment me. The monster who raped will always

remain there, to haunt me, if not in physical reality in the abyss of my thoughts.

A slave! Why didn't I die?

I looked at myself, naked on the bed, and I felt ashamed as this body that betrayed me. Then I moved away from the bed, hastily I put on my trousers and top and prepared to leave the room. I went downstairs and found myself in the studio. Gino was there, sitting on a chair smoking a cigarette. I avoided his gaze for I could not face another humiliation. At length I was out of his studio, away from that degrading experience. Francine, I said to myself. You must die.

I wept till I had no tears to shed. My whole life had been ruined, and I had no glimpse of what the future could hold for me.

That night I stood in front of the mirror and looked at my distorted image, observing the once beautiful woman, now fragmented with dark shadows. If only she could stop, but she did not heed my plea, for the other Francine remained there, staring at me, reminding me of the calamity which befell me. And I could not take it anymore, no longer.

But what could I do? Even, the breath inside me betrayed me. Finally I managed to sleep, for it is there that I long to forget my devastated, shattered reality.

SHATTERED WINGS

Two days after that distressing incident between me and Gino, he called me again. Gino expected an explanation, or perhaps he would like to understand my situation, but I could not confide in any other man. Nor could I face him again after what had happened between us.

So, that was another milestone in my life, and the absolute truth was that my life and fate were overshadowed by one single event which my mind could never conceal. This reality was slowly, slowly wrecking my life.....

I went on along the path of life, existing rather than living. My life at home, at work and with my friends continued to flow. I was still clinging to the mask I d' constructed for myself to keep away the pain. It was all a cover up. It felt as if I was on a train, sitting, exhausted by the voyage which led to nowhere. Yet, I kept going on my voyage to my unknown destination, where the only hope was death.

Death did not come, as if to defy me, to watch me suffer, agonising in my yearning to be taken by it. This was rather strange, for the Angel of Death only comes to take the innocent, the pure; what contrast to me! I thought of Stephanie and of Juan. The thought of that poor boy sends tremors all over my body. He was not like his father. Not at all, and it was only through my work that I found the courage to go on. A new hope was instilled in me and this time my journey was heading to a remarkable encounter.

That was Erika.

At times the rays of the sun peer through our windows and induce us to embrace them. It did also for me, and the rays of sun shone into my soul. My encounter with Erika was a gift from God to show me that I was not stumbling alone into this path of sheer devastation. Rape, though a silent crime is universal amongst us women and this reality was a stepping stone towards my healing.
Erika, who was admitted in our ward for further investigations, came from Bosnia and was studying psychology in Malta. Erika must have been in her early thirties. She was a lovely woman, with long chestnut hair and beautiful blue eyes on fair skin, but her eyes were rather sad, revealing the hardships she had to go through during the war in Bosnia. Her English was also good, which made it easier for us to understand her. I liked her accent, which was present whenever she talked.

Like all other patients, I gave her the best attention she deserved and she took the opportunity to talk to me about the war in Bosnia. I was flabbergasted with what she told me about the war and in my heart I thanked God that I was living in a peaceful land. That seemed to relieve me a bit. Erika told me that she had to flee from her country to escape the hardships they had to endure. Confronted with the pain and calamity of others, I managed to reappraise that part of myself who had endured the pain and suffering of sexual violence.

Later on, I was to discover another aspect of rape.

SHATTERED WINGS

Erika's results were normal and there was no indication of serious illness, so she was discharged from out ward, and before she left she approached me.

'Miss Francine, I would like to thank you for your help,' she started by saying.

I held her hands firmly and looked into her eyes, and it was there that I could sense the grief and pain which their gaze demonstrated.

'I hope we won't see you again here,' I said.

Her eyes were penetrating mine.

'But I hope to see you again, perhaps, in some other place.'

I smiled at her.

'Yes, why not,' I remarked.

'Come to the convent where I live,' she said, handing me a sheet of paper.

'I'd love you to come.'

'I will,' I said, and helped her out of the ward.

In the days which followed I kept thinking of Erika. Her words confused me. I knew there was more in those sad eyes. So, I made up my mind and went to meet Erika again. One fine afternoon I found myself knocking the door of the Sister's convent. It was September, and the fierce heat of summer was fading. We were looking forward to the autumn, but I was heading for another revelation.

A small nun opened the door for me.

'Yes,' she said.

'I would like to speak to Erika,' I said.

'Who are you?' she asked me again.

'Tell her it's Francine.'

The nun led me to a small room and I sat down on one of the chairs. There was peace in this place and for the first time I felt a sense of peace entering me. The stillness of the place permeated my soul and I longed to remain here, away from my burdens. Then my eyes fell on the crucifix hanging on the wall.

My God, where were you when I was violated that night? I thought. I got no answer, but only stillness which I could not understand. I preferred not to think as my thoughts were already burdened by the past.

A familiar voice brought me back to reality.

'Hello Francine.'

I looked up and saw Erika.

'Erika!' I exclaimed.

I stood up and embraced her.

'Thank you for coming, I knew you would come, I felt it in my prayers.'

Prayers, I thought. I looked at her bewildered.

This woman prayed and I had forgotten all about prayers, even the existence of God.

'Come, would you like to go in the garden?'

'Oh yes,' I replied.

I followed her into the garden. It was a huge garden and the stillness which I felt previously in the room was still lingering here. I took a deep breath to embrace the pure fresh air. Erika looked radiant, even though overshadowed by pain.

We then sat down on a bench under a huge tree. She looked at me smiling.

SHATTERED WINGS

'How are you Francine?' she asked me with her eyes looking deeply at me.

'I'm fine, and you?'

'Now that you have come I feel happy.'

She took my hands and held them firmly.

'So you are staying here.' I said.

'The Sisters' offered me shelter while I continue my studies.'

'So you will be going back?'

'It will take some time. I might work here, but in the meantime I want you to help me.'

I stared at her, bewildered. How could I help her? I was still recovering from my trauma, at least I hoped so. What Erika was going to tell me was indeed far more devastating than my experience.

Erica's eyes looked at me sadly.

'I know you can help me, you are warm and kind.'

Everyone said this about my eyes, but they also concealed a lot.

'You are confused, let me tell you.'

She paused, for a moment silence stood between us, but in that silence there were noises and screaming of a soul who wanted to be heard. Erica spoke again and looked directly at me as she started her story.

ERIKA

In 1992 Bosnia Herzegovina declared its independence from Yugoslavia. It was then that the Yugoslav Army, along with Serbs nationalists launched the war in Bosnia Herzegovina which was ethnically mixed. It led to endless days of ethnic cleansing.

At that time I was living with my sister in Bosnia, our parents died a year before, and I had nowhere to go. My sister, who has lost her husband in an accident, had asked me to go and stay with her. I did not hesitate to accept, as moving with her helped to relieve the pain and void left by my parents. The village was surrounded by countryside and high hills, and I loved the simple life in the village. I was eighteen and was looking for a job while helping my sister. All was well until the war broke out and the magnificent hills and the evergreen areas were turned to Hell and we women were the ones to pay for this sacrifice,' she explained and continued, 'It was a dispute between two territories and it led to this senseless war. This was more of a cynical battle between groups with one single aim; to grab as much territory as they could. These were years of Hell, but the most frightening were the measures the Serbian army used as a form of ethnic cleansing for eliminating us, the Bosnian Muslims. Soldiers were all around. until one day they showed us what they were made of.'

SHATTERED WINGS

Erika stopped and lowered her head, then looked up at me and her eyes were drowning in tears.
I held her hands, Erika's lips formed into words.
'Then the worst thing happened. One day I went shopping, it was still daylight and so quite safe for a girl. Or so I thought. I put on the veil and went out, as that evening I was going to cook a treat for my sister. I had been walking for ten minutes when an automobile stopped. I looked and it was the military. I kept walking, trying to avoid them. We had heard about the Serbs, but I could never imagine that they could go so far,'

Erika looked at me as tears started to roll down her face, 'The car stopped and the soldiers came out of it. I kept walking, but they were following me. All of a sudden, I felt a pair of arms gripping my shoulders. It was them, the soldiers. I was petrified and tried to think if I d' done something wrong, but it had nothing to do with me. One of the soldiers grabbed me and took off my veil. Then with his hands he stroked my cheeks, 'What do you want?' I asked him, full of consternation.

He did not answer but he grabbed me again and threw me on the ground. I tried hard to release myself, but it was all in vain, he was stronger than I was. Then he covered my mouth and with the other hand he went through my garments looking for my thighs. I cried and I knew what he was up to, what he was going to do with me. He was lying over my body and I could feel something on my thighs. I've never been touched by a man and did not know what it meant,' her whole body was shaking with the memory.

'He continued forcing his thing inside of my thighs and then I felt great pain, as if something hard was entering, deeper and deeper and to a certain extent, killing me. Then it occurred to me that this was rape. It did not end here and more was to come. I made an effort to move, but they did not let me. More soldiers came down and one after the other they took their turn in raping fiercely one after the other. Their laughter echoed around in the air, and I heard one of them murmuring, 'She is a virgin, and men do not get them everyday.' I can still hear his voice now. Then I heard another one saying loudly; 'You will raise your bastard as Serb.' Then the men laughed loudly and left me alone on the ground.'

Erika stopped, her tears now pouring. I remained dumbfounded. This was hard to believe. Like me, Erika was introduced to Hell; she was brutally raped by these monsters, in an ordeal probably far worse than mine. Her story took me back again to my experience, but in my pain I felt a sense of belonging with her.

This woman received my full admiration. She could talk about her experience, whilst I could not.
Erika was watching me, and then continued with her story.
'It was extremely hard to stand the pain. Being a Muslim, our virtue is of utmost importance. It felt humiliated, and deprived of any dignity. I just

wanted to die, but there was my sister, yet when I arrived home a horrible scene was awaiting me. This scene will remain forever engraved in my mind. I recognised the car at once. A shiver ran all over my spine as it suddenly occurred to me that the soldiers were there. No, this could not be. My feet felt clumsy, but I plucked up my courage and walked in the house. There I witnessed the greatest shock of my life. The most horrifying scene was before me. This was far worse than the rape and I could not believe my eyes. On the cold ground my sister was lying in a pool, drowned in blood, whilst a Serb soldier was doing up his trousers. I thought I was going to faint and my feet were paralyzed. I stood there, motionless, staring at the scene, dazed as if I was an alien. I could not register the fact that my sister was lying there, lifeless.

Suddenly I felt sick, terribly sick and fainted on that beloved body. I do not recall it all, only images. In a flash of a second, visions of our childhood came, where both of us were playing together. Little did we know how we were going to end in this way, Then suddenly, I felt a pair of arms taking me away from my sister s' corpse. 'No, no,' I sobbed, for I wanted to remain with my sister, to die with her; but there was more for me. They were taking me away, and I looked at the one who was carrying me from the hand. I shuddered. He was a soldier, and I can still remember his gaze. His squinting eyes penetrated me and pierced my heart. More soldiers came in and dragged me off with them.'

Erika stopped again and covered her face with both hands, but then went on, her eyes fixed on mine.

'Francine, it was not enough they wanted more from us. The Serb Soldiers dragged me by the hand and forced me to walk. 'Where are you taking me?' I asked one of the men. 'You will soon know.' Devastated and wretched as I was, I dared not utter any other word. The soldiers were huge and looked hard and I did not want to go through the same experience. Yet, it was to that experience that I was heading again. So I kept walking, barefooted, and even if the ground was rough, it did not damage me as much as the previous scenes. Yet, I kept walking and walking, even though my soul has left me and perhaps even life, until they ordered me to stop. We stopped near another village where other women joined me. We looked at each other, but could not talk. I could easily grasp the truth behind their harrowed expressions, full of grief. We were merely lost souls, walking and walking away from our homes which once warmed our hearts. After long hours of walking we arrived in the countryside area where there were large buildings, and we were forced in the place.' Erika took a second to steady herself and wipe her tears.

'I found myself in a large hall, with only beds, and there were other women who stared at us, with the same appalled looks. There was no life in their eyes and all had been taken from them. These women were just waiting for death, and soon I was to be like them. Now, that my sister was gone, my honour defaced, there was nothing left to live for. Most of the women were pregnant, some in advanced pregnancy, others in their beginnings. For a moment, I felt like being driven into Hell.

I went to sit near a woman who was in her late forties. Her eyes were dark and had dark circles under her them, her cheeks were slanted and firm, revealing her beautiful high cheekbones. The woman looked at me and said in a low voice. 'It would have been better for you if you died my child.' In that horrid darkness, I thought of my sister. What a way to die! Yet, she had been right, for what was following was far worse than death. Looking back, I say that I would have preferred to go with the flow of death, rather than going through the events which followed. Certainly, the hands of God were with me constantly.'

Erika looked me in the eyes once more, they still glistened with the tears, 'The Serbs were responsible for these camps, and later I learned the reason why I was in the camp, the same reason for the other women. These camps consisted of stores, empty factories and old schools, and all served the purpose, to accommodate the Serbian soldiers in their tasks of eliminating Bosnian women by raping them. They referred to it as ethnic cleansing. We were the victims. Then it was my turn. A man wearing a uniform in his late thirties took me by the hand. 'What do you want from me?' I asked him. He grabbed me and threw me on the floor. A sudden prickle ran all over my spine for I could tell what was coming. They were going to rape me again., 'Open your legs!' he shouted using these hard cold, words. I tried to resist, but he untied his trousers and came closer. I fell onto the ground and suddenly he was all over my body. His filthy body was penetrating me, then there was a searing pain and he was raping me fiercely, another officer entered in the room. I took a deep breath and sighed with relief as I thought that they were going to stop. But this Hell was not going to end; it was only a change from one soldier to the other. The nightmare was to go on, for the other soldier took down his pants and raped me. There was no way out. I closed my eyes and lost consciousness. When I opened my eyes I found myself in a dark room. Then it all came back and it suddenly dawned upon me that I was a prisoner. From the other room I could hear screams of other women. These women were of all ages and were being raped like me. Why was this happening? What were they taking from us? It was dark in the room, with only a dim light to help us see, but there was nothing to see but pain and misery, which overwhelmed us. I heard the door being opened. No, not again I thought. My limbs were aching and I felt weak and was not ready for another assault,' she wiped her eyes with her sleeve.

'No,' I screamed and covered my face with both hands. This time I was going to resist them. Someone entered in the room, but they were not soldiers. Instead it was a six year old girl. She walked in and went to hide in a corner. Even though it was dark I could still see her skirt stained with blood. The girl sat opposite me and stared at me and then burst into tears. I moved from my place, sat beside her and stroked her cheeks, but she hit me. I knew she wanted to remain alone, but my heart was torn into pieces for the deep pain she was experiencing. A six year old girl, not even a woman! What did she do to deserve this? Why all this? I left her alone and went back in my place but my heart was prostrated with grief. That night was an endless journey to Hell and I lay awake, recalling what all the scenes and what I went through. Images of my sister's lifeless body came before my eyes, and then the wretched girl facing the wall.'

'One after the other, women came into the room and only the walls can recall the tears which we shed in silence. In the darkness and in the stillness we have forgotten the meaning of being a woman. With each new day we hoped that this would come to an end. It did not. We were raped by military Serbs every day and no women escaped their barbaric lust. They used to tell us they had orders, but I knew the reason behind these actions, they wanted to humiliate us, to lose our honour because we were Muslims. Most of us were virgins in times of rape and we gave away our innocence to these savages. Moral shame was the deepest wound, as for us premarital sex is prohibited, and yet they came and took it away. I gave my innocence to someone who did not love me-not a man but a savage. '

'The rapes went on as a punishment, but we were exhausted, devastated and destroyed. There was no life left. We were under control. Some of the women even died, the others were walking ghosts. Then my periods stopped, and it was not due to shock, but the repetitive rape by them monsters. I noticed that my belly was expanding and this was not due to overeating, we ate very little. Along came the nausea and the illness, and there was an instinctive deep feeling which warned me. I was pregnant. Being raped is already a nightmare, but carrying an unwanted seed is a grave reality.'

'Who was the father? It was not easy to tell, as there were many of these savages who brutally raped, ravaged me, for how many times which I dread to recall. There was life inside me; a child who was innocent. We remained in the camp for more days and even months and now, there was no doubt of my situation. I was with child, but being pregnant did not alter our situation, and we were still subject to rape. The soldiers went on raping and raping. In my memory there is a horrid scene which will never leave me, a scene of a pregnant woman in her eight month. I saw them, the soldiers, raping her one after the other until she was exhausted, till she could no longer breathe. But what could we do?'

'With every new dawn we hoped that this would be over. Instead we were over, driven from our families, our villages. The only comfort and strength we found was in our company. The affinity in our tragedies was what kept us together and the love and solidarity between us kept us going. We lived day by day, because our body kept breathing, yet every one of us prayed and longed that our souls travel with the night. They did not. One fine day it was again my turn. I went for a walk, from the filthy smells of rape, away from the place which was beginning to haunt me. I walked, but a soldier was walking behind me. Even in broad daylight these were men without scruples, who attempt to rape us in every situation. He grabbed me. I could not tell which one of them it was, for every time there were new ones. Now, rape had become a daily part of our life, shattering our hopes and making us immune to everything. I tried to escape, but he seized me. He brought out a knife and put it close to my throat, so close that I could not breathe.'

''Do not dare resist me!' he said in a harsh voice. I knew there was no escape. Then I thought of the child who was growing inside me. They could not kill me, for killing me would take away my child, and for the sake of my child I let myself be raped again. It did not hurt me anymore, as rape has become a part of me, and for the first time there was a mission, a purpose embodied with this evil act, and while he fiercely penetrated his body inside me, my sacrifice was being offered for my child. There was nothing to live for, neither to die for. We have become mad machines. Then one day all this stopped, but we were already lost and lifeless. The harm done by Serbs will remain engraved in our minds and in our souls. We will always recall that silent cry in the night. It will always be there.'

'We were taken to see a doctor where most of us were in a state of shock and had infections. I carried on with my pregnancy. I wanted to carry my child, even though many other women with similar situations asked to abort their child. I have lost everything, but there was this child growing inside of me. Though ashamed of myself for losing my virtues and my dignity, I wanted this child. There were times when I thought about my days in the camps and saw them acting like beasts. Thinking that one of them was the father of my child was a chilling thought which pierced my heart. In the long nights I cried and cursed myself, but my child had nothing to do with all this. Inside of me there was a new life and all I could was to it protection. Carrying their seed in my womb day after day was an ordeal, and there were moments when I thought I would have a monster instead of a child. Soon, however, I discarded these thoughts and went on.'

'If the worst came to the worst I could give my baby up to adoption. I had a choice; to abort the child and finish with it, but I was alone in the world and needed a child, however it was conceived. Also, the pregnancy was already in its advanced stage, and it was not right. The child would sense the pain. Yet, it seemed that this child sensed everything and for an unknown reason has decided not to come into this world. Perhaps it sensed the coldness and darkness of my experiences, or knew how it was conceived. So, the child decided to desert me. After, long days of waiting, I gave birth to a still born child.'

'I still recall the dim light in the cold delivery room in hospital. The pain and the forceful movements were to no avail. My child did not make it. The sweet voice of the nurse trying to soothe sounded in my ears like the monstrous voice of the soldiers who raped me and killed my child. Francine, I wanted to keep the child but fate was hard, very hard.'

Erika stopped and covered her face with both hands. I embraced her, trying to control the emotions which flooded all over me. Her words brought me back to my own reality. Suddenly, Erika's story opened a new gate of more memories where the scenes came before my eyes. In my visions George appeared again, and I pictured him forcing himself inside me, then I was again on the coach, waiting to abort. It all came back and like a film I visualised all that I have been through, but pregnancy after rape creates more pain and misery, inflicted both on mother and child. This thought brought comfort in my heart. At last, after coming across this woman, who like me, had shared the same fate.

Then Erika went on.
'It took me ten years to start living normally after the trauma, but my life was doomed. I went back to my village, but I was a different woman, torn with thorns of life, burnt in the ashes of war. No, man could enter in my heart now, nor did I dream of one. With therapy and counselling I managed to start living again hoping to leave behind me the trauma. Yet, when I close my eyes every night, the image of the six year old girl comes to haunt me, as if to remind me of the constant nightmares we had to endure one day after the other. I often wonder what has become of her. Is she still alive? Does she still recall the constant horror she had to constantly

endure in silence and drowning in tears. As for me, I can still see her hiding away in the corner, her skirt soaked with blood. One thing is certain, that this scene will remain inscribed in the chapters of my life. Yet, God never leave us threading alone in this path.'

Erika stopped and stared blankly at me, her eyes drowning in tears. A long silence reigned between us, and in the stifling atmosphere our thoughts were combined in one single train. Face to face with her story, I felt overwrought with this overpowering experience of Erika and her people. I could not utter any single word, the reality of rape is too hard to grasp, for I was already reliving it again. All I did was to hold Erika's hands firmly whilst trying hard to hold back the tears which were spurting from my soul. Sitting beside me was a lost soul like me and I thought of Christ on the crucifix. Now I knew he was living in this young woman. Yet, I shuddered at the reality of men, but what kind of beasts were we dealing with? How could they do it?

Erica was one of the few women who survived and it suddenly dawned upon me that I too had survived. There were others, sisters and perhaps brothers, who did not survive, who did not make it and could not bear to face their truth. These were the victims of ethnic cleansing, where rape and violence were utilized to dominate a nation, mostly on women.

I sighed. Yet, I marveled at how our paths had crossed, she coming from different land, different culture. There must have been some divine plan, both of us took the same journeys of shame, of physical, emotional and psychological humiliation, suffered in full awareness, in the depths of our souls, where no one could hear our cries. The invaders made us shed the silent tears, which could only be heard by those who are thrown in the same journey, like my sisters, the thousands of Muslim girls and women who endured rape; those who did and did not survived.

For the first time I was no longer alone, hiding beneath the facades of oppression, but there was a new courage being rekindled within me. It was God who answered my cries by sending this woman to show me the truth. There was stillness now between us, which was restoring our lives. I put my arms around her and then Erika s' lips formed into words.
'Thank you Francine, I feel much better now.'

I embraced her again and in this warm embrace I felt like finding a new sister. Even I was feeling better, and it felt like releasing a heavy burden from my heart. There was a new dawn which had come for us. This new light was reflected in Erika's eyes, which all the sadness and pain ebbed away, and even my heart felt lighter; as if two souls have rediscovered each other again. That was the final realisation that we were not forsaken.
'You have been through a lot, my dear,' I said tenderly.
'Now it's all over and I am here, but I have more to tell you, if you have more time.'

'Yes, of course,' I replied. I did not want to leave her, but to remain with her for all the time.
Erika gripped my hands and uttered in a low voice.
'Thanks, Francine.'

So, she continued with her account of her afflicting suffering. After losing her child Erika went back to the village and tried to settle there. It was hard for her as there were too many memories to remind her of her tragedy. Erika was destroyed, lost and alone, but with therapy and help she managed to get her pieces together. Her courage returned and got a job and went on with her life but, this was not enough. Erika wanted to do more. The shadows of pain and the harsh reality of misery made instilled within her the need to help others. This was a blessing. She would never forget her past or the sufferings of her sisters which she shared with them. Then one fine day a new path was presented to her, an opportunity which she could not refuse. This was a scholarship to follow a course in Psychology and that gave rise to a new chapter. Erika had a good knowledge of English and adequate educational background. She was offered an opportunity in Malta and now she was in her final year.

The corners of her mouth smiled, releasing the pleasure and relief she was experience.
'Now you know my story. It's the first time I am talking to someone about it since I came to Malta,' she said softly.

SHATTERED WINGS

I stared at her bewildered. But why choose me? Perhaps she sensed that I had been threading the same path.

'You can count on me,' I replied, demonstrating my deep feelings. The tears were streaming on my cheeks, but they were tears of release. After, many endless months I found the courage to come face to face with the truth of rape.

Erika spoke again, holding my hands firmly.

'I know,' she murmured, 'God led me to the road of thorns to help others, people like me who went through the same experience.'

I could not but marvel at this woman's faith and courage in dealing with this situation. Compared to her, I could not even face myself after what I have been through. Just a moment before, I could not face the man on the Cross, but this woman still retained hope. As for me, the act of rape had given birth to a murderer who lived inside of me.

Erika went on, 'Through my studies, I found new ways to help me comprehend the situation and even conquer my fears. Of course, this was not easy, especially when I read about the psychopathology of the rapist.'

The word rapists sent tremors all over my body, reminding me of their horrendous acts and even thinking of them made me sick, but I plucked up my courage and asked her dismissively.

'Do you think they are ill?'

'Not all of them I must say, but there are some cases.'

I thought of George and the brutal soldiers. Could they be ill? No, they were rather driven by their inner urges, compelling them to invade us, invade our velvet. Yet, I wished that George was ill, that he was somehow unable to control his impulses. Perhaps that would have altered my perception. Indeed, I would see him in different light and who knows, I would be able to forgive him.

That day would never dawn in my heart.

Erika must have been reading my mind, for she said, 'I know you do not agree with me, but we have to find a way to help victims and reduce the incidence of rape.'
How could we stop them? Her words baffled me and I could not grasp the meaning behind them.

Surely, she had something on mind which I could not perceive, due to the intense emotions aroused by this savage word which overshadowed my past and governed my present. Erika was unaware of what was passing from my mind; she did not know that I had been raped. To her I seemed the strong, dedicated nurse and I was in doubt if I should tell her about my experience or not. It was better to keep it buried inside of me.

I heard her say, 'It's ok Francine, if you come and see me tomorrow afternoon at university I will show you a project.'
I stared at her, confused, and I thought that I did not hear right, so I said,
'A project?'

SHATTERED WINGS

She nodded, and for a moment I felt thrown into a world of confusion, I could not figure out what she had in mind. Could it be a project for them? The ones who rape and violate? Then I would have to cancel everything and cut the ties with her.

'What project?' I asked her again, but I did not get an answer, which added to my curiosity.

Erika said in her calm voice, 'I will explain everything tomorrow. Is it fine with you at university?'

So she was not ready to tell me, but I wanted to see her as being with her felt good, like a light in the dark. Erika was sent from heaven to accompany me and to help me emerge out of this long dark passage leading to an unknown destination which I could not bear to foresee, and yes, I promised to meet her at university the next day. Her eyes were beaming as she held my hands firmly.

'I am happy,' she said in a low voice, 'So until tomorrow.'

That was agreed. Then it was time for me to leave her. I kissed Erika on her cheeks and left her place. I walked away from the convent, my steps slow, but steadily pondering, almost overwhelmed by Erika's experience. For the first time, I felt peace in my heart, as if my parts were becoming together at last.

Finally!

The night which followed took me to a succession of thoughts and images. Sleep evaded me and the night was already decided for me. I laid awake, thinking, reliving Erika's story. I pictured her in the camp amongst other women. I saw the soldiers raping them mercilessly. It was like a film before my eyes, Erika's angelic face being stained by lust and fouled by the breath of a savage. It was brutally hard, an unimaginable nightmare which horrifies and forces us to close our eyes, to not to see these heinous atrocities inflicted on those who were most vulnerable. But they were real and hovering with us, haunting us to make us face them, one day. I did, for I was there, as were Erika and the other women. Not only the women, but also children and men. A chill ran all over my body as I recalled Erika's recount. I pictured the six year old girl. My God! How could they do that to a six year old girl, tearing her apart? Even for a grown up it was painful. In the darkness of night I conjured up the scene of her being raped, the hard wood forced inside her, a little girl. Tears were my only consolation, tears of pain and desperation, as if I was the girl herself. In the deep darkness of the room I could see it clearly as if I had been there. Her imaged cries permeated my soul and echoed in the tunnels of my mind.

Bastards! They took away her innocence and now she was wrecked in a life which abhorred her. Then I thought of the days when I was her age. At that time I was falling in love with the Temples, introduced to their mystery, whilst this little girl was being introduced to Hell and delved deeper in the flames of men. If only I could embrace her, but she was far, far away, yet so close in my thoughts. She will always remain with me, along with that night, and the shadow of George.

Then again the soft image of Erika came before my eyes and her constant fortitude gave me new hope, lighting up my heart and instilling a new belief. It appeared to me that the dark gloomy thoughts engraved in my mind by the devastating experience of rape and the loss of love were fading away in the fog, at least for a while. Overshadowing my life, there was only the reality of Erika and other women like her. We were all sisters and bruised by fate, yet we could easily comprehend our sufferings and perhaps even open a new road to recovery. Alone, I have crossed the dark path, for days and nights without seeing the light. Now there was a new candle which promised light out of the tunnel.

Our roads were parallel and now there was a project awaiting us, even it had yet to be unfolded. With these thoughts coming and going, sleep came to visit me but this night was different from the ones before it. It was free from the usual nightmares and the memories of events which often come to visit me. There was something to look forward to, and I knew that there was no way back; only walking forward towards the light. That night was casting a new light, as if the moon changed its gown and was dancing with the stars. It was also in her dreams that Francine met her other part and could look into the mirror again. In her eyes she could see freckles of light, stars shining in the brown mingled with green of her eyes. They were smiling, full of hope. Erika was this hope, the new faith.

There was another day where the first signs of dawn brought a new perspective in my life. Even though I slept very little the night before, I was feeling good and refreshed, prepared for a new day, a new horizon. As planned and as configured by fate, that afternoon I headed towards University in order to meet Erika. I had no idea about her project or what she wanted from me, but I had complete faith in her. And yes, an inner force urged me to help her and my feet compelled me to go. There was a new force which lightened my heart, as if my life has changed overnight.

Perhaps, my prayers have been answered, my cries had been heard and a new page in my life was about to begin.

University was unique and exhilarating; clusters of energy mingled together. It is where students live, study and share their aspirations and dreams. I walked by the campus area where students were all gathered, laughing, chatting and discussing. How I longed to be one of them! There were students of all ages, but they were mostly young people. I walked amongst them and with every step I could sense their zest and energy for life. That was the contrast between us. I was young, but I could not look at the future with their eyes. We had different paths, but at the end of my walk there was hope waiting for me.

SHATTERED WINGS

The canteen was not far, I walked in where Erica was waiting for me in a quite corner, sitting alone at the end of a bench. She saw me at once and waved at me. I kissed her on her cheeks and sat down beside her.

'Hi Francine! I knew you would come,' she said with her eyes beaming.

'Of course.'

'It means you are interested.'

Even though I had been in the dark of this project and totally unaware of what it entailed, I could not wait for Erika to tell me what she was proposing. As it was afternoon, the canteen was almost deserted, as most students were having lectures. This enabled us to discuss in ease and in complete tranquillity.

Erika was watching me intently, and her eyes were soft and smiling.

'So, tell me about the project.'

Erika smiled, 'I wonder what you might be thinking, that we met only for a while and I am asking you to help me.'

'No, not at all. It seems that I have known you for years.'

'I too had the same feeling.'

This was indeed real, there was an affinity between us and the more I looked into her eyes, the more I felt her close to me. We were two souls, perhaps finding each other after the dark tunnel.

What Erika was proposing left me dumbfounded, but not with grief or shock like in previous days. Though overwhelmed, I felt a sense of relief, as if doors were being opened for me and I thought it was another dream.

Erika's mouth formed into words, 'Francine, as far as I know there is no specialised centre for victims?'
Her words astounded me. No, there were services, but no centres.
'No,' I replied, but my mind went back in time. I thought of the day when I was raped, at the police station and the shame which overtook me as I spoke of my experience. Perhaps, if there was someone to help me, to guide me, then my story would have been different.

Erika continued, 'This is the project we need to set up.'
I could not believe her and for a moment I thought this was a dream.
'You mean a centre for victims of r-?' I stopped abruptly, for I could not utter the word, but Erika went on.
'Yes, for victims of rape.'
Her voice echoed in my ears like beating drums. This was a noble idea, but it was too much for me but for me. Where did we have to start? Erika must have been reading my mind as she said, 'Perhaps, you were not expecting this. I know, but we must work for the victims and put pressure against the rapists and these types of offenders.'

This woman's vision was beyond measure, based on great courage and I admired her. This woman, who was a survivor of a Hellish nightmare, was thinking of her life and wanted to help other victims, like myself. But could we do it? From where do we start? My eyes could not see any path other than that of living day after day and waiting for the direction to be unfolded. Violence had blinded me and made vulnerable and feeling lost. On the other hand, I knew that something had to be done to stop violence.

The burden was for us to carry, we who were introduced and engulfed in the darkness of violence, somewhere we returned to with every breath. Back we went to face the lust in our perpetrators eyes, but the idea of the project was slowly setting in the corners of my mind.

'Erika,' I said, 'how are we going to start?'

She sipped her coffee and kindly offered to get me some; I had been immersed in what she had to say. Then, she brought a pile of papers out of her briefcase.

'Francine, these are my ideas.'

I stared at her at blankly.

'Don't tell me it's about the centre?'

She nodded.

'I did it while I was in my first year of studies. I know, you're thinking, how did I manage all this?'

'No, far from it,' I interrupted, bewildered for I could not believe the fact that she had got this far. She was still there on the threshold of suffering, and yet, showed was an ocean of infinite strength.

I was amazed at the contrasting reality between us. Rape had left me weak and disjointed, but meeting her had made me whole. My soul had finally found itself and embraced the light.

Then Erika handed me the documents and told me to read them, which I promised to do. After I had read her Idea's, we had to meet again and discuss. Erika looked at me and her eyes were smiling. The sadness in which I have read in her gaze, the first time I saw her seemed to have ebbed away. There was only light, reflecting her inner peace. Love had come to take place in that dark wounded corner of her heart. She did it and so had I. Yet, in my hands I was carrying this light, which not only unburden my heart, but that of others who were still waiting in the dark.

My mind was overwhelmed by these pages. They promised new life, and I could not wait to start the journey through them, as if all of a sudden I had a new companion. A different companion, who would not rape me and reading through the first page was giving birth to a new beginning. There was a new chapter which was folding with the others, yet this chapter was predestined to move the curtains out of my heart.

Then, I quickly looked through the window, in which I could see the faint light of the sun rising, and my heart was lifted. Each page, each line was inscribed by sweat and blood, retelling the story entwined of the devastating breath of a woman running away from her shadow. I went through the pages, detail by detail. In the document Erika wrote about the services which could be offered to victims of rape. In the following pages she described in full detail the process of the reporting of crime, until the court proceedings. This was a procedure which I had missed and I wonder how many women went through it. It was shameful to report the crime of rape, as there were many stages to take. The lack of understanding from others humiliated victims of rape. There are people out there who think that the woman deserved to be raped. Perhaps, the way she was dressed or behaved. This is totally out of context, for a woman who is more daring in her dress attire or a woman who flirts is not asking for rape, but for attention or other reason. Rape is an act against the woman's consent and no should be taken for a no.

Another factor was that there were other women who were not wearing provocative clothes or involving themselves in a seductive manner, yet still had been raped. There were victims of war like Erika and even bedridden women and patients in institutions.

The worst moment for the victim would be when filing criminal charges against perpetrators. Any thing could happen. The pages which followed stressed on the importance of the medical examination, which had a special interest for me, as they came from the field of nursing. Through the examination swabs, the evidence of the crime is contained and can later be presented in court. Another fact was the occurrence of pregnancy and sexually transmitted diseases. The victim should be given the choice whether to continue or not with her pregnancy. I stopped and thought of my experience. A sudden prickling ran all over my spine when I thought of my ill fate, of becoming pregnant after rape. It is at this stage that the victim would be needing help. Being raped is already traumatic and the incidence of pregnancy and these same pages took me back to the days of my pregnancy. It was utterly hard where I was embodied in a crucial situation which baffled me and left me astray with my fate. With the burden of sudden pregnancy overshadowing me, I was given no choice. Abortion was my solution, but I had taken the life which was dwelling inside me. Perhaps, this was not the best solution, but was there another way? Erika too had lost her child, but in different circumstances, yet, our children shared the same ill fate of being conceived from the breath of violence. Promptly, I went to the next pages where Erika continued writing on the needs of these victims. Most of all, victims of rape need to be aware of every step taken, which concerns them and this is better attained by professional people. This entails constant support from the moment the victim is raped, until the criminal proceedings in court.

Erika wrote on how victims face their perpetrators in the same corridors in court. Most offenders go to court with their family members and friends, and for the victim, this creates terror. Thinking of ever having the opportunity of coming face to face with George made me shudder. His presence would remind me of what he did to me and in his fierce gaze would rape me. How could I give my testimony in his presence and of others? How could I retell, detail by detail the humiliating force he imposed upon me, his forceful entry in my body.

Of course I could not face him. Seeing him again instills deep within me feelings of strong aversion and revenge for I detested him. Yet, many victims are still going through this experience, facing their aggressors, testifying against them and recalling with precise detail what they had to go through. This is another trauma, where victims relive their afflicted episode again. That was indeed real and I totally agreed with this concept. Erika went on stressing on the importance of providing support at this stage. Yet, it was amazing how this woman despite her distress and her trauma came up with these ideas. I marveled at this document which brought to light the real sufferings which victims have to go through.

This was the beginning of a project, but like any other road it had its prices. For me, the papers were the beginning of my second life and I owed this to Erika.

In my heart there was new hope which slowly, slowly was dawning upon me. Understanding the pain and misery of others at times adds in the process of healing. Erika's concepts had to be manifested and I had to live to see the day.

Another dawn took its turn like it does every day. For me, it meant more and gone were dawns which promised no light where I wished they had never come. Now the sun was shining again. The following day Erika was waiting for me at the entrance of the library at university. I approached her and kissed her on her cheeks. This was the moment I waited for. Erika looked at me, her eyes full of questions. I knew she could not wait for my views about her writings. We walked up the stairs and headed for the large hall engrossed with large shelves of books. I sighed as we walked by these sections. There were books on every topic waiting for students to take them. They were life's companions and I thought about how much I loved to read before and immerse myself in books. Now, they were here to remind me of their presence and what they promised. There were days in my life when I dreamt of studying medicine. That was still a possibility and the shelves seemed to convey this new belief. This was a miracle, a new birth, but now there was the project ahead of us.

In a solitary corner, near the window, there were two empty chairs and we went to sit there. The library was deserted today and we could easily talk without disturbing others.
Erika broke the silence.
'So, what do you think?'
What did I think? That it was a great project which overwhelmed.
I gripped her hands and caressed them.
'It's remarkable, with so much detail. I never thought.'
'I know. It took me three years of work and research.'
'Since you were here,' I retorted.

SHATTERED WINGS

Erika lowered her head thoughtfully and then she looked directly at me.

'Francine, the experience of rape has changed me. I can never erase from my mind what I had to endure. No day passes without me thinking of the event. Maybe it's not so strong, but the memory is still there, but I've read that the best way to heal is to confront the situation and do something about it. And that s' what I did.'

Listening to her talking felt like waterfall crystals permeating my soul. Her courage inspired me and filled me with a new courage, the will to live. And now this remarkable woman wanted to help others with this interesting project. The sparkling light in her eyes whenever she talked about her project instilled within me new life. I loved her as if I had known her for years.

Erika spoke again, 'I would say that rape is the sister of death, but I did not die.'

No, we did not die and we were here to do something. Her strong words echoed in my ears. Then I took her hands again.

'No, they did not kill us.' I heard myself saying.

Erika looked at me, puzzled, I was expecting this reaction from her, but the time had come for her to learn about my experience of rape. Sharing with her ordeals, her tragedies opened my heart and incited me to talk about my rape. This was the first time I had spoken about it, after almost one year.

I plucked up my courage, looked at her and said, 'I've been there too,'

Erica looked at me with tenderness in her eyes, 'Oh, dear. It must have been hard for you. You are so nice.'

Her soft words touched me. Suddenly all the memories came before my eyes and George was again before me as if he had taken her place. A sudden prickling ran all over my spine and I felt a lump in my throat.

No other words could come out of my lips, exactly when I decided to talk about it. That is because I could not talk about it, as the memories were so deeply buried inside me that they could not emerge now. That was more painful. I saw her moving from her seat, come close to me and put her arms around me.

'I understand,' she uttered and her voice soothed me and opened my heart.

'Francine, I know a place where we can talk.'

Erika took me by the hand and led me out of the library. We walked in utter silence, but our minds were overcrowded with thoughts. Yet, at the same time my heart was relieved, even if it was only one word which opened up to a new understanding.

In the depths of silence there was the new seed of healing. But the thought that I was in good hands made me feel safe. For the first time after the rape I felt safe. Hand in hand we walked, leading each other to our next path. Our steps took us away from the crowds and loud voices gathered all in the Campus area, but the chattering noises of students did not affect me now. In my heart there were outcries and loud noises waiting to be heard.

SHATTERED WINGS

We finally arrived in a tranquil place, secluded and at the end of the university buildings. There were trees and some benches around. I presumed this was an ideal place for those students who sought some peace. Today it was meant for us. I felt at ease in this place and was attracted by its stillness, in harmony with nature. From afar, I could hear the soft humming of the birds and for an instant I envied them, happy and free. What a contrasting reality to mine? Yet, the silence of the place and the genuine beatings of the heart in the woman sitting beside me lured me. I felt drawn to the warm blue eyes watching me. Step by step with all the details I recounted my experience to Erika. For the first time I talked about George, the rape and the abortion, whilst Erika listened emphatically to my story. In her warm look full of love and compassion I felt peace again. Tears streamed on my cheeks, but these tears were more of an appeasing nature. I heard Erika's angelic voice saying these words, 'Believe me, I could tell that you have suffered in life. Yes, I could see it in your eyes Francine, they are warm but sad, but now I am here for you.'

'Thank you,' I rendered and then embraced her.
Erika went on, 'Well, if you reported him, it would have been different.'
Then she looked at me and paused.
'No, I understand your situation. Being an important person and would have made it difficult for you. He would have gone away with it.'
I sighed with relief. At last there was someone who echoed my thoughts, and now the veil of guilt had been lifted.

'Francine, now you can better understand why the centre is so important for victims and those who get raped.'

She was right, and in the perspective of my past events I appreciated the need for the service, Erika was proposing. Yes, in my case, if I had got help I would have proceeded against him. But I was threading alone in a dark, rough road leading to definite collapse. If there was someone walking with me, like Erika had walked with me, then it would have been otherwise. Then, George would have been brought to Justice, and he would not rape again, not me nor others. But that was far from truth. Yet, at that still moment I enjoyed visualizing George being locked in prison, suffering deep humiliation. Deep down I knew that day would never dawn.

At the moment, there was Erika, whose similar fate and warmth gave me a new birth and took off the burdens which overhauled me. A new sun was rising and there was only one road ahead of us. That was the project where Erika has put all her life, her hopes in this project. Perhaps like me, but in other way Erika was also suffocating her pain and drowning in her reality. It did not really matter as long we walked together and whatever it was, what kept her blood throbbing in her veins, it kept mine too.

Erika held my hands firmly.
'We will see the sun again.'
'Yes,' I added, 'and we will open our hearts again.'

SHATTERED WINGS

Love! Did I really believe in love? The truth was that I had ceased to believe in it. In an instant the images of Ivan and Gino came before me. I recollected the moments of complete innocence with Ivan and then the tenderness of Gino, which I could not accept. My heart grieved for the latter, for I have lost him, all because of the shadow of raped. I felt a pang in my heart as I thought again of these shadows casting all over my consciousness. Well, love may have deserted me, but it lived in Erika s' warm gaze.

And I followed her light.

Confiding in Erika changed my life and promised a new dawn. Having already met her was a breakthrough in my life, but sharing my story with her strengthened my path. Now, we looked forward for the project to materialize, and one way or the other we had to arrive. Our predators arrived before us and we could not let them override us with their everlasting greed for lust and power. The result of this was violence with the aim of destroying us. Erika had been right; they did not kill us. We were survivors and this was what made us strong enough to work together on a new project which was the beginning of the end.

The days which followed were hectic, where we had to move from our dream and start working. Setting up a project entailed lots of work and research. I must say, the more I read about rape the more I felt myself emerging from the past. And through all our efforts, we were heading for a miracle. We kept working on the project by adding more detail to the document. Along with our work we got versions from the police, from lawyers and other caring professionals. This brought us to the fact that such a center was needed on the island, even though there were services which provided help for victims. This was not enough and our conclusion was that there should be a specialised centre with specialised people to help victims of rape in each and every moment of their trauma. The effects of rape do not stop at the time one is raped, but start after the crime, remaining with the victim for almost a lifetime.

But most of all I regained my freedom, and this was attained through working with Erika, which filled me with sheer determination to go on. Other days came to haunt me, which brought back memories and regrets, but this time I could not look back as there was a road awaiting us and slowly we were heading for it.

That was the onset of our healing.

The research on the proposed project took us almost three months; quite a short time, but we worked constantly. For Erika it entailed more effort, for she was in her final year of studies. Yet it seemed to me that the divine hand of God was leading us. Perhaps, I thought, God was making up for the sheer cold dark moment when he was hiding beneath the clouds. That was a dark day which inscribed the brutal word in the corners of our minds. Now, it faded and before us there was only this miracle.

When we finished our work I just I could not believe my eyes. Here, before our eyes, there were loads of papers weaved on our pain and that of our sisters in every part of the world. That day was special and we were University, precisely in that quite area. This had become our best loved place. This place meant a lot to me, for it was here that I was enchanted by its stillness and the petals of my heart were opened again.

Till the dawn of truth.

Tears rolled down on my cheeks and then I embraced Erika. She too was moved, but was thoughtful. Then she looked blankly at me. I gripped her hands.
'Erika, what's wrong?' I asked her concerned.
She smiled. 'Nothing. Well, I am thinking of my people, my sister and the other girls.'
I fully comprehended her thoughts. Erika was contemplating all the scenes, the events which she had to go through. I pictured the women being raped day after day, their screams echoed in the void. It was all in vain. Their eyes had become like holes with no expression. This would never be cancelled from her memories. Never.

I shuddered. Again, as the image of the six year old girl who was with Erika came in my vision to haunt me. This project was for her. Yes, but where is she? This single thought tormented me, but I

Marie Anne Zammit

preferred to look at the other soul who was with her, that night.
'I am sorry for your people,' I said faintly.
Yet, gazing in those eyes did not conceal my images, in fact there was more. Visions of the Bosnian girls were coming before my eyes. When Erika told me about them I was shocked, dumbfounded, but now I was seeing everything, as if I had been there. Yes, I pictured the Muslim girls buried in their virtues, then being strapped and humiliated. Death sounded sweeter than tasting the cold-blooded lust of the savage soldiers. Then there was their seed to carry. The pregnancies and burdens imposed on them. They were children reproduced in seeds of hatred and violence. What world awaited them?

All in all, women's power was insulted, and the goddess inside us was again deflowered by patriarchal beings. It is sad, so sad, this reality veiling our lids. I knew that at this special moment Erika was back in her country, passing through the passages of her past. Yet, our future was giving us a new child and this was created on the seeds of love, unlike the others who were the result of a tragic night. They could not come to the world and turned back along the dark long tunnel of existence. Our children had to go. Erika's baby died by accident, mine was a different story. I was constrained to remove it, to shred it into nothingness. But then I would have detested it, just as I detest his creator.

SHATTERED WINGS

It did not really matter. Surely, God would understand the pain in a women's heart. Yet, here was another child waiting to be born and heard. Well, the truth may be residing with us that men will always rape, that there is nothing to stop them, but we were strong enough to combat the effects of their deeds. We were helping victims not to remain victims. That was a long way ahead. Seeing our work coming to completion created a moment of intense emotion for me and Erica. It had been her idea and was reaped on the winds of despair.

I hugged her and kissed her on her cheeks and said with a firm voice, 'If we managed to survive all this, then other women will follow our steps.'
Erika looked at me, her eyes full of tears.
'Yes, we survived,'
The warm rays of the sun reached us and were slowly, slowly casting their shadows on the trees. Magnificent scene! At that moment I wished I had been an artist, then, I could capture this beauty.

This thought was soon overshadowed by another one, as I thought of Gino. He was the only man whose memory I recall with tenderness. He was not here and would never be, but I did not want to think about loss today. No, I wanted to embrace this moment. This moment under the trees was real, magical and liberated from every thought or emotion which taunted me. In this real moment I only longed to watch the sun, bestowing its rays on the leaves. And the trees never seemed greener than that day.

I smiled and the color of the leaves permeated my heart.

Now that we have come to the first step there were more to follow and we could not leave it for ourselves. We needed the help of other professionals to give us their views and Professor Borg, the consultant in the ward where I worked was the next person to see our project. I knew I could trust him and that he would be interested. Indeed he was, and he asked me to see him in his office. I kept my appointment and on one evening, after I finished work, I headed up to his office. Professor Borg's presence made me feel at ease, as he was calm and considerate both with patients and staff.

He looked at me behind his spectacles, while I briefly described the project to him. He then watched me intently and his warm gaze behind his glasses comforted me.
Then he spoke, 'Well, Francine, this sounds interesting.'

Professor Borg paused and my heart leaped. I wondered what he was going to say next. Waves of trepidation ran all over my body. What if he rejects my idea? Then I had no one to turn to. But what was I conjuring up; I let my thoughts take over my mind.

Professor Borg was speaking again, 'Francine, I will read your proposal and then if you would like, I will offer my suggestions.'

SHATTERED WINGS

I stared at him bewildered but my heart was overjoyed.

'Yes, of course. Profs Borg. I said, 'You mean it can work.'

'Yes, but let me go through it.'

'Thanks, Professor Borg,' was all I could say and then prepared to go.

Professor Borg gripped my hand and held it firmly.

'Francine, you have my full support. You know I always knew you would do something great.'

I blushed, but his words filled me with joy.

'I am not alone in this. Good day Professor Borg.'

Then I went out of his office, elated. With Professor Borg's help the project would thrive and come to its succession.

Deep in my heart I knew that we were heading in the right direction. It was our re-birth and the way out of our traumas. My meetings with Erika were more often where we shared our emotions.

There were no regrets for divulging with Erika my story, which like hers was weaved on pain and surpassed by male virility. Now, life appeared much easier. Both of us were walking away from the deep grief which clouded our hearts and dwarfed our thoughts with those devised by our villains. There were news waiting for us which conveyed faith and hope.

Three days after my meeting with Professor Borg, he sent for me. The hours before the meeting were filled with anticipation, where I waited eagerly for this meeting. I wondered what Professor Borg had to say about the project, but something inside me told me that positive news awaited me. I went in the office where Professor Borg was seated.

He asked me to sit down which I did, then he looked steadily at me.
'Francine, I read this document and I must say you've done a very good job.'
His words made me feel good. I sighed with relief. That was the first step. Professor Borg looked at me thoughtfully, while his hands went around the pages lying before him.

It was our document. He was speaking again.
'What you have written here is necessary and important, but I am concerned.'
Professor Borg paused and looked again at me, and I wonder what was next.
'My views are that this project is rather complicated and involves a lot of departments.'
I knew that, but we had to start from somewhere. With his firm voice and kind heart, Professor Borg explained to me step by step what we had to do. One suggestion was approaching people from the media and inviting them to write articles on the subject and discuss it in detail. That would create awareness and more people would be interested. As from his part, Professor Borg promised to help us in writing to the Authorities concerned. A wave of excitement swept all over me. I could not believe that this was really happening and with the entire support of Professor Borg we were going to succeed. We have already started, but the road was not easy.

SHATTERED WINGS

After my interesting and fruitful meeting with Professor Borg I went down to the ward and called Erica to tell her the news. From her voice I could sense her joy.

'This is wonderful, Francine,' she said. 'I know some one from the press who can help us. I will call you again.'

'Ok, my love,' I murmured.

A feeling of exultation swept all over me, but I tried to restrain myself as there was work to do. One thing I was certain; Francine was finding herself again. What followed was not complicated. We managed to get people from the media and one journalist accepted to interview us. Her name was Marion, a young attractive woman who worked for an independent newspaper. Erika was supposed to be there, but refrained at the last minute as she was feeling rather uncomfortable, so I accepted to go in her place.

Marion was understanding and grasped the topic immediately. She did not stay back from discussing the debatable issues of abortion and the morning after pill. For sure, these will create endless controversies, especially in our Catholic community. But this was not going to stop us from expressing our views, regarding these subjects. Strongly, I believed that women in case of rape should be given the option to decide whether to keep the child or not. If at all possible abortion should be avoided.

Throughout the interview, we mainly focused on the silent grief which victims of rape have to endure, along with the traumas, the fear and the pain. Finally, how victims can be helped. I could easily see that Marion liked our idea of the crisis centre and stressed on the importance of such a centre. Overall, the interview went very well, arousing the interest of others making our cries heard.

A new beginning was dawning upon me and Erika and soon we were going to bear fruit.
Two weeks later the article was on the press and I felt proud of myself. Proud that I had found the courage to do what I did, whereas some months before I was contemplating death, struggling whether to keep on living or die. I did not die for life sent me Erika. As I went through the pages I could not hold back the tears which streamed all over my cheeks. These tears were sweet, conceived from seeds of joy as the tears of desperation; of utter sadness were dissolving, ebbing away in the light of our project.

But, my journey was not yet completed.

The article was even read by my colleagues at work and the day after when I returned everyone was congratulating me for the interview. Most of all, they were all backing the idea and this filled me with joy, a new wave of happiness strengthened me. Then I thought of Ivan, and felt a pang in my heart. What if he was here, what would he think? But then, I thought if he was here, my reality would have been altered. Then, I would not have been raped. But he was far away, and far from my heart, for now there was only the project which took over me, my life.

Yes, the project was our life. More months elapsed, during which we worked hard to accomplish our goal, to fulfill our dream. There was more work, more interviews and greater awareness. Seeing our idea taking new life came as a surprise to us, but we tried to enjoy every moment of it.

Indeed, we had every reason to be amazed for there were many other people who were showing interest in our project. Amongst them was Victoria, a young lawyer who joined us to help us in the legal aspect of rape. Others who came were teachers, social workers, psychology students and even victims. For us, this was our greatest achievement, for reaching victims was our target. Once victims get over their traumas, once they talk about it and admit their pain and tragedies, they become survivors, and in surviving they discover that they are no longer alone, but one pearl in a string of pearls.

That was our strength.

Janice was one of the pearls who wanted to join this string. She approached us, to share with us her experience. Janice was twenty five and was having psychiatric help. This lovely woman had heard about our project and wanted to help. Janice recounted how, on one night after closing her shop where she worked as a salesgirl, she was heading for the most terrible experience of her life. As she was walking away from the shop, heading for home, a car stopped and the man driving offered her a lift. At first Janice did not heed him and kept walking, but the man insisted and Janice thought he was being kind to her. It did not occur to her what she had been heading into. Janice accepted his lift and went into his car, presuming he was genuinely going to drive her home safely. He did drive her, but he had other intentions in mind.

He was not going to drive her home and changed his direction at once. It did not take long for Janice to realise that he was taking her to the destination he promised her. Suddenly, he stopped the car and Janice consummated her reality. She found herself alone, in a remote area, in a place under construction. No single soul visited this place. Politely, Janice asked him to take her back, but he told her to wait as he was going to keep his word. Not before he got his way. To Janice's utter surprise she saw him taking off his trousers, he was naked from the waist down. He moved closer and Janice was astounded to see his private part close to her face. She thought she was going to faint facing this disgusted situation. He was adamant in getting what he wanted, besides there was no way out, Janice was locked in the car, alone with this monster wearing the mask of a man.

Then his penis was near her lips and he forced her to put it in her mouth, forcing her to perform oral sex. Janice attempted to resist him, but this was to no avail as her resistance added to his lust, increasing his drive. Momentarily, Janice managed to move her head away, but then the reality descended upon her like cold shower. She was locked alone with him and anything could happen. Indeed she was right, he then brought out a small pocket knife from hid shirt and put it closer to her throat and intimidated her, threatening with her life. Janice had no choice. So she had to do it

Then he attempted to do it again, and with no resistance to hinder his impulses. He had won the battle, as Janice having no choice conceded to his demand. The poor woman had to endure his forceful, unwanted disgustful act. Like a famished, sexually depraved monster, this stranger grasped Janice's face and brought it closer to his thing. Janice, against her will, constrained by terror and consternation had to do it.

After he finished, he let her go. She was devastated, overwhelmed and full of trepidation, Janice managed to leave the place and arrive home. The only person she could confide in was her sister and she helped her to report to the police.

The man was brought to Justice, but this did not alter Janice's life. No one can bring back her peace and security she lost that night. Janice is now another woman, overshadowed by her past. For her, men are monsters who are there to grab her and abuse her, use her like a toy. In the same instance, Janice feels intimidated by men and cannot trust them. Above all, Janice is afraid of riding with them again. It was only through counseling and professional help that she is finding herself again. Today, Janice strongly advices other women against accepting lifts from strangers for no other reason.

These women who came to confide with us their experience of rape and sexual assault strengthened our will to go on, and empowered our project.

Jennifer was another young woman, who after hearing of our project made up her mind to approach us. It was hard for her to relate her experience with us. I could appreciate this after she told us her version, which shed new light on what was actually happening in certain circles.

What was supposed to be a party ended up in a nightmare of unpredictable events, ending in rape. I would say that Jennifer's story brought together some of the pieces of my life. Jennifer was twenty five and in her final studies in Commerce and Management. She told us how on one night she got an invitation by Mark, one of her male friends, to attend for a party. Mark was in his early forties and a manager of an established business firm.

The party was held in a large villa, and for Jennifer this was an opportunity to meet people from the field and to establish contacts for her future. The people invited were business men and people in high society. Amongst them there were Members of Parliament and others in high positions. I shuddered as George came in my mind. The reality which Jennifer recounted to us was appalling, yet unbelievable, and I found it hard to register that this in fact reality. She was enjoying the party and stayed till late. Not many people remained and the ones who stayed were nearly all drunk.

Jennifer was having a drink, chatting with one of the guests when Mark came and grabbed her by the hand.
'Are we going so soon?' she asked him. Mark did not answer, but kept walking dragging her behind him. He led her through dark corridors and then upstairs. Still, Jennifer could not conclude what was happening. At first glance, she thought this was a joke but what followed was no joke.
Another man approached her and took her by the hand.
'What is this game?' she asked him.

Again she got no answer, but she recalls the man covering her eyes and mouth with a black cloth and then dragging her inside a room. Someone was helping her and leading the way. Jennifer found herself on a soft mattress. It suddenly occurred to her that she was laying on a bed. She struggled to release herself, but it was all in vain as she was encircled by men. They were so close to her that she could smell their breath, reeking of alcohol. One of the men moved close to her, so close to her that he was almost lying on her. Then, he started to fondle her breasts, moving his hand all over her body. Jennifer attempted again to release herself, but this seemed to increase the man's ardent desire and forced himself inside of her, leading to rape. He started moaning and uttered some words which she did not understand, some nasty word referring to his state of utter sexual ecstasy. I could easily reckon that state where men lose their reasoning when lost in lust and passion. The stranger's voice was rather familiar, but in that moment Jennifer could not associate it. All, she wanted was to get away from this trap she found herself in. Jennifer cried and pleaded with them to let her go, but this accentuated their passion. Then they were finished and left her. She was relieved, and though she was feeling weak and in stupor, she tried to move away. Again, she did not succeed for another man came and made her lie on bed and raped her again.

This was more than she could take, but Jennifer had no choice. When it was all over they left her side and locked her in the room. For hours Jennifer was left alone in bed. She took off the cloth and tried to get some rest, if she could get any. It must have been night now, but Jennifer was only aware of the dim light in the room and the haunting memory of the previous experience. It suddenly dawned upon her that Mark had betrayed her and that this was not a party at all, but there was something grave going on. There was no time to ponder about that. Jennifer was kept prisoner here and the worst could happen. She already had fathomed that she would not come out alive from the room. It was an inkling which tormented her and disturbed her sleep. Then someone opened the door and Jennifer saw a masked man entering in the room. She shuddered. She knew what to expect now. They had come to rape her again. The man grabbed her by the hand and led her out of the room. The light in the corridor was hurting her eyes but what followed was far more serious. The man ordered her to keep silent and threatened to kill her if she mentioned any single word about this party.

Jennifer was compelled to suffer in deep silence. She feared for her life, but did not escape the harsh effects of rape. As a consequence, she failed from her studies and attempted suicide with no success.

Jennifer's experience was similar to our story, in which, for most of the time, silence is our river which keeps us flowing. Yet, what Jennifer related about the people present at the so-called party, made me seriously think about George. Could it be he was part of it? A sudden chill ran all over my body. Well, anything could be. According to Jennifer, this formed part of a secret society where men could freely express their sexuality without the restraints of everyday social life. That was one of the reasons why, amongst the guests, Jennifer recognised certain people in high positions. In this secret place all inhibitions would vanish and this was a great opportunity for these men their fetish desires and perverse fantasies.

Most of these perverse desires included rape and any other form of sexuality which deemed pleasurable at the moment. Learning about these deviant thoughts and inclinations revolted me. These men were sick, but also very well protected and their secret guarded. It will remain safeguarded until their victims speak up. Jennifer was one of the victims who decided to address this problem. After two years of keeping this secret within her, Jennifer decided to share with us this serious fact. We had one thing in common; the silence which protected our secret and of those who hurt and degrade us with their uncontrolled lust and passion. We were all emerging from this silence, which for years had suffocated us. No, not any longer.

There is a saying, if you help yourself, then God or the Universe will follow with its help. This was indeed true. The days which dawned upon us were full of rays of sunshine which filled our heart with more hope. Hope and success presented itself to Erika's path as she got the results of her final exams. Erika passed her exams, completing her studies in Psychology. It was a great day for her, for us. There were tears in her eyes, tears of bliss which lifted the sadness from her eyes. I was overjoyed and could not hide the waves of elation which flooded all over me.

We embraced each other and our in our heartily embrace we voiced all our emotions which could not be expressed, but our hearts and souls had already grasped it.
'We made it together,' Erika said her voice full of emotion.
'Yes, and you were the light of my life,' I added.
'No, the light in our hearts simply met.'
We walked together under the clear heavens above us. They were watching us, protecting us and showing us the way. In all my life, never have I

seen the sky so clear, crystal blue, reflecting in Erika's eyes. The light was our project which had to lighten the hearts of other victims. It was where it was most needed and they were going to get it.

I marvel at times, at the turning points in one's life, how that seems to be glowing can fade the next day. All in all, what is beautiful always carries a price behind it. I paid the price, but the subsequent events made me even stronger. Our plan was finalised, yet it dawned upon me that my road was not yet clear from the shadows of the past. It did not take me long to grasp the reality which was surmounting me. It occurred to me that someone was following my steps and like a cold shower descending upon me, this notion entered my head.

Amongst the days which came to bestow the rays of the sun upon us, there was another day which did not bring the sun. This was the day when I got the first call. This was the first of many. It was a normal day like others and I was at work one of my colleagues called me to tell me that I had a phone call. I felt overjoyed, presuming that this was from someone interested in our project, I ran to answer the phone. But I had been wrong, very wrong.
It was a man s' voice who spoke on the line.
'Are you, Francine?' I heard him say.
'Yes, how can I help you?' I responded.
'Miss, let us come to the point at once. Take this warning seriously. Stop the project.'
I was stunned, and for a moment I thought I was in a bad dream again, like those bad dreams which used to haunt me night and day. Well, it seemed

that they were back again. What intentions did he have? And who was he?

'Sorry, but I cannot understand,' I faltered.

He was persistent in his senseless threat. I heard him say.

'Another step and you won't live another single day. I warned you now.'

'What warning?' I asked him, but he cut the line.

This unexpected and mysterious phone call left me speechless. I remained motionless, staring at the ceiling pondering on the call, which baffled me and left me stranded. Back in the staff room I kept thinking of him. But what was this? Was I reverting back to the dreaded past but this was reality. There was only the voice echoing in my ears, overpowering my thoughts and I felt descending in a long dark narrow tunnel, with no signs of light. While alone in the room I tried to recall the voice. It was a strong, harsh voice which was ringing in my ears. The voice was utterly new but surely the motive was contrived by a familiar aim. What was definitely true was that there was a single soul or more, perhaps who were against this project. I thought I had an inkling of who this man was.

In one instant moment I found myself in the past, the place which a moment ago I thought I have lost with the winds of fate. It had returned again now.

My nightmare was initiating, and this time I will not win.

SHATTERED WINGS

My peace, which was regained with the previous events, was suddenly shattered and faded away with the occurrence of this call. No matter how hard I struggled to eliminate this episode, it was still there. Even the dim colour of desperation overcrowded me and my soul was transported back to the old memories. This event was destined to go on.

Whoever had called me was adamant in not letting go, as he called again, two days later, with the same warning. But why me? The answer was in my heart.

Yet I tried not to heed these calls and kept on with my work and hoped it would stop there. They did not, for he called again, the same words, the same time. Now, there was no doubt, but I kept it buried in silence. My life had taken a twist. Now there was a wave of fear overshadowing my life. Now my steps were being scrutinized by someone whose sole aim was to deprive victims from their freedom, and who could it be other than those who create them with their scrupulous vices and violence.

The menacing threats of the phone calls managed to take me back to the endless path darkened by fear, but did not stop me from working for the project. For the sake of Erika and the rest of the other women, the secret had to remain entombed with me. Surely, a thing like this would upset them and demoralise their dream of seeing the project taking life. The secret was for me to keep, to protect my sisters. Yet, my days were full of consternation, where I kept wondering who was this man.

I feared of what could come next and this filled me with trepidation.

Our project flourished and there were more people, mostly women, interested and who came to join us. Our meetings took place at University or in public places, but soon we were going to have a place. At least, this served to alienate me from the recent experiences and seeing this filled my heart with joy and strength to go on with it.

Then all of a sudden, the intimidating calls stopped and I felt relieved for a while. Indeed, it was for a while for it did not take me long to note that I was being followed. This was after one of our meetings. I noticed a car following me while I walked to the bus stop. The first time I did not really worry, for in the area surrounding university sometimes you get sad cases' that goes there to pester young women. Yet, when this kept re-occurring, it made me ponder seriously on his presence there. I thought of the calls and now I had no single doubt that he was scrutinising our steps. I shivered, for if I kept seeing this mysterious man at University that would mean that he knew about all our moves. This included also our project. So, they knew about our steps.

Then, a shiver ran all over my spine as I recalled Jennifer's story. She had taken a risk by confiding in us, the horrid experience of rape. Most of all, Jennifer uncovered their sacred secret which could not afford to be revealed. And George was one of them and George had raped me.

Perhaps they knew about our moves towards our goals, but we knew their secret. The latter had serious implications.

Notwithstanding all these elements, which came to disrupt our plans, we kept on going, working on our goals. Victims could not wait no longer; they had waited for too long, where every minute seems like eternity. The journey after rape is a long dark trail and the victims are the ones who suffer in deep silence. Nightmares become their sole companions and the memories of rape appear more lucid than dreams. It almost feels like having a dual personality and suicide becomes the ultimate solution to alleviate the sorrow and desperation, leading to a dramatic end where death becomes the mistress of the play, creating a poetic verse to annihilate the soul. I had been on the edge of this act, and I wondered whether I was heading for another one. There are victims who never end this journey and find themselves stuck in deep abyss of darkness. I knew this route by heart, as I had been threading its road, but now that there were new steps ahead of us the journey was part of the past. The victims did not wait any more.

There was a day when the rays of the sun reflected on their faces. This was the turning point when the project which we suggested as Rape Crises Centre was presented to the Minister of Social Affairs. I was happy, but there was an underlying fear that George would intervene. Well, yes, in his position he could use every measure to stop us. Perhaps, he already did and I thought of the telephone calls. No he could not, I reassured myself to banish the staggering thoughts which were already tormenting me. He could not stop us, not now that our message was clearly delivered. The rest was in God's hands.

Days turned into weeks and then months. The warm days of summer again started to heat our days, but we were focused on only one aim. During these long, endless days we waited eagerly for the outcome. Deep in our hearts we knew that the project was in its way to materialise. We could not let go now, as our mission had been completed. This was our new dawn. Yet, I was still tied to the past. This came as a shock to me, for I thought that I had supervened the past. This truth came through a dream. One night I dreamt of a man seizing me, trying to rob me. He opened my purse, but he did not take my money, he tried to kiss me and then forced himself inside me. In the dream I shouted, but my voice could not be heard. Then I saw George's face. I woke up, startled. My hands were clammy and my body was sweating. The dream was so real, so vivid that it felt like suffocating me. There was no denying it, the memory of George was still buried inside me and it came to taunt me and humiliate me.

It will always remain there, walking with me with every step I take. Looking at my hands reminded me that they were stained with blood, the blood of my child. Suddenly, all the memories, all the events came vividly before me, as if it has happened the day before. My heart felt heavy when the thought of my child re-appeared again. George had made out of me a murderer out of me, I killed my own flesh and blood.

I hated him to death. But why this endless struggle to forget the rape? Just when I thought that I had survived. The worst realisation is that the struggle against rape is against my own self. It was utterly hard to accept that reality. These thoughts remained with me until the early hours, along with the light of the moon entering from the window. The moon was waxing; paying homage to the Goddess, but that night it wasn't looking at me nor listening to the faint rhythm of my heartbeat. I was alone with myself. Then I closed my eyes, hoping to be invaded by sleep. To my relief the image of the project came before my eyes. And this comforted me.

By autumn we received the first response. It was good news, as if fate was in conjunction with the steps of nature. I was breathless and a feeling of exultation swept all over me. Well, the project was accepted and was going to be funded. The dream was becoming reality. There were many experts who were expected to give their contribution in order to implement a strategy.

The Rape Crisis Centre was going to operate on a twenty-four hours basis. Once a rape had taken place, the victim would go to the centre or someone would go and explain to her what was next. Should the victim decide to report the rape to the police, she will be then advised about all the procedures which follow. Also, the cultivation of evidence was important and would be used later in court.

During medical examination the victim will be accompanied by some one from the centre. She would then be tested for HIV and pregnancy. Yet, this was going to be a dilemma. What if she gets pregnant? In Malta, there were no measures such as morning after pill. Given the circumstance of being hit by pregnancy, the victim concerned will be given counseling to help her decide what to do with her child, if possible to find ways to live with it. Yet, she should be given the choice and respect to decide what is best for her life.

A great day was ahead of us and that was the inauguration of the centre. The centre was officially inaugurated by the Minister and there were other people from high authorities. At first, a feeling of apprehension overwhelmed me as I thought of George. I feared that he would be there. No, this could not be. He was far too wise to present himself, but there was no doubt that he knew what was going on. This did not bother me. Today was a special day for us, what we had waited for, for so long was reality. Amongst the people who were present there was Professor Borg whose constant support never ceased.

Proudly, I stood watching the scene, full of emotion. Erika was standing close to me. I looked at her and I could see that her eyes were full of tears. In that moment of bliss, Erika traveled back to her past, where thoughts resided in her homeland, still under the shadow of the devastating war.

But today there was no place for tears, we have cried enough. Now it was time to rejoice, for reaping the fruits of our endeavour.

The night which followed brought me peace again. I looked at the moon which, though waning was still corresponding with the feminine spirit within me. The battle against my thoughts had been conquered and after many days of utter darkness and void I felt whole, away from that fragmented personality I had to bear for days and nights.

Then I closed the window, and unknowingly my feet led me to the mirror, and the woman looking back smiled at me. I smiled at her with the same smile which I gave her in her childhood, during her studies and through her work. Then I stopped. I thought of love, of Ivan, and the feelings of sadness surfaced again. This disappointment may be etched in the corners of my mouth, but what mattered today was that Francine was smiling again and tears were streaming on my cheeks.

What followed was exactly what we had envisaged in our project, and we had been right when we said that more people would report the crime of rape. The centre and the services encouraged them to report and the process was working very well.

For us it meant our mission was done. Erika had applied to be part of the professional team and she was accepted. She was overjoyed and I had no doubt that she was one of the best. I owed her a lot, for she was the first step towards my healing away from this journey. Erika was also the first stone of this centre which brought us hope. We were really blessed to be in the company of a strong woman. Erika will remain in my heart forever for she was the one who walked with me and helped me to look at the stars, the moon and the sea again.

And that made me live again.

The centre was functioning well with every professional giving her or his contribution. Erika too was happy and looked radiant and her eyes regained their smile again. We were happy and satisfied with the outcome, for the centre was serving as companion in the journey away from rape. Victims were now on their journey towards survival. Yet, we were not aware that there were other individuals who were dismayed and feeling uneasy with this centre. It was inevitable; more victims were reporting the rape and that meant that more perpetrators were being brought to justice, taken to court and sentenced.

This gave reassurance to victims that they were safe, at least for a while till they are in prison. At least they won't do it again.

Or will they ?

SHATTERED WINGS

Reporting them and testifying against them is an ordeal and no easy task, but on the other side of the coin it empowers victims. The fact that a victim had the courage to do something makes her feel responsible over her life.

It takes courage, which I did not have, but I admired the women, children and men who could do it. Rape and sexual assault should be reported immediately for this ensures that they are deterred. For me, they are inhuman, monsters who demonstrate their powers and virility by inflicting pain on those who are vulnerable.

Little did I know that one of these monsters was close to us, closer than we could imagine. And while we were giving all our energy and our life for the centre, which was our creation, someone else was contriving a plan to destroy it. I could not believe that they could come to such length. Yet, they did.

Another nightmare has begun, and slowly, slowly, it led to the end of my journey.

The next day which dawned was created on threads of evil and darkness. This darkness brought us face to face with reality with our adversaries whose sole aim was to demolish and break down our centre. It would have been better for all of us if it never dawned at all for this day took us back to our misery, to our pain which we sought to conceal from our memories.

Most of all, the victims were deceived, flabbergasted by this poignant act. Yet, nature is a cycle which we dared not dabble with, for it was far too dangerous and we had to admit that we could not change it. And that was our staggering truth.

Seasons come in cycles, one ring leading to the other, like life. These cycles in life appear in the form of a journey, like clouds passing swiftly on the ladder of our souls. Then, all at once, the facts unfolded before my eyes like thunderstorms freezing my bones.

I saw it happening, yet it was unbelievable. This shattering episode which collaborated with the past was hard to bear. It made me ask if it was real and if it was really happening to me. This time was rather different, as my question had been answered. We too got our answer. It was a direct answer which left us all naked and alone in the storm which hit us without warning.

Well, I'd had warnings. The savage truth hit me and threw me into an abyss of desperation. Every trace of hope was now diminished, lost with the wind, which unknowingly dragged it away. Suddenly, darkness plunged upon me again, and again.

And I had been there before.

The news astounded me, like and it felt like being hit by a fist. I could not believe my ears when it Erika called me at work and told me that someone burnt the centre.

SHATTERED WINGS

Our centre!

'Francine,' she said sobbing, 'The centre has been burnt.'

My god! I was stunned and stared blankly at the wall, for a moment I thought I was in a very bad dream. I asked her to repeat again the words, but I had heard the right words. My heart was racing now and I thought I was going to faint. Could this be true? Erika's voice echoed in my ears.

'Yes, Francine, last night some one entered and burnt the first floor, there was no staff.'

I could hardly utter any single word after learning these devastating facts. Erika asked me to see her in the afternoon and I agreed.

Suddenly all the courage and hope were forlorn and I could see no other way out of this dark dungeon. Before this odious action I had no strength and who did it had won. I sat down and stared at the ceiling, my vision was blurred, yet, still there were images which came to torment me. The centre, our project was destructed and it felt like being raped again. The tears which rolled on my cheeks could not stop now. Then the truth dawned upon me.

Jennifer's experience came to mind. I recalled her story, her mentioning of the secret society. Could it be that they were involved in all this? Then there were the calls, the threats and warnings. All this was concocted- but by whom? Perhaps, I had an inkling of who was the author and doom fell upon me. A sudden prickle ran all over my spine. That was the end for me and I could see no other step forward, no future.

It was all over and even fate had forsaken me.

Still not believing that our centre had been burnt, that afternoon I left early from work and went straight on to the place. I hoped that it was not so bad, but when I arrived on the spot there was a horrid scene which was hard to bear. The staggering reality pierced my hearts like daggers. The buildings were completely destroyed. Panic seized me and had to hold Erika s' hands.

Professor Borg came to join us and the three of us stared, numb at what had remained of the centre. Everything around us was stained, and there were only traces of smut and the intoxicating smell which suffocated us. It did not matter now; the centre was completely destructed, shred into nothing.

The tower which we had constructed was now ashes and I did not know when this Hell was going to end. Then, I thought of the long hours spent working, researching till the end, till we brought our dream to reality. It was all in vain and all perished with the wind of hatred and revenge.

I had the same feeling, which altered my destiny. I stood, motionless, watching the ruins felt like I was going back in time to where George was. His cold eyes were looking straight at me, scrutinising me, waiting for the moment to act. It was evident now that his shadow was overpowering me again, especially on this day where he has won. Suddenly, I felt a pair of hands around my neck. No, no, he was close again but it was not him.

I sighed with relief. It was the hand of an Angel.
'Erika,' I heard myself hearing. She looked at, her eyes glistening with tears. I held her hand firmly.
'Why, did it happen, Erika, Why?'
Erika did not answer, but lowered her head thoughtfully transported back in her past. We were both there reliving our misery, but even confronted with this misfortune and the shattering of our plans, there was no time for self pity.

Erika looked up at me.
'We will go on Francine, we've been worse than that.'
Yes, we have been worse than that, but the centre had passed through the hands of our aggressors. I did not utter another word, but stared blankly. Yes, we have been through many voyages in our past which led us to this. Yet, I could not help thinking that our child had been murdered and our souls raped again.
'Yes, we will go on,' I said firmly.
Did I really believe these words?

Deep in my heart, hope had forsaken me, left me bereft and all the walls felt like collapsing upon me. But, then looking at Erika filled my heart with courage. I could not leave her alone in this road which was ahead of us. Professor Borg's presence helped to comfort us from the feelings of desperation and helplessness which was taking its toll on us.

Six months has elapsed from its inauguration and the centre was destroyed by villains. Nevertheless, I could not configure up the reason why our centre was the target of all this aversion. We were doing nothing wrong, but then we were helping women to report their crime and these men were exposed.

Perhaps, there was another reason, and this was more the probability. We knew their secret which they tried to conceal. And that gave us power over them.

All the media were talking about the centre, giving it prominence on all front cover. It made it worse for me, for every report reminded me of our failure or better, our misfortunes. There was going to be an enquiry to detect and determine the cause of the fires. It was going to take a long time, but at least we were going to get response. I had no doubt that this was vengeance and the thought that someone, in some other place was celebrating their triumph, tormented me.

While we descended into utter darkness our enemies were content, threading their paths in silence and their sins tarnishing their souls.

One day this would end, but when?

Though discouraged and utterly bewildered by this incident, we were determined to go on. During the months which followed we waited anxiously for the report. Still, there was no final conclusion from the enquiry and it was going to take long. Well, there were many factors to be considered. An inner urge propelled me to speak about the strange calls which I got some months before, which helped to throw new light on the investigations. It was apparent that someone wanted us out of the way and there must have been a very serious intent. It was far more severe. While we waited for the report, the women and the professionals kept meeting where another temporary place was found to accommodate victims.

No violence could stop us from attaining our goals, once we started we could not go back, even in our hearts we were feeling dejected. For my part it seemed that there were more lessons to learn, as these realities never cease to daunt me. At times I wonder why I didn't let myself go with the waves that night. It would have been a different story, but then Erika would have not met me and the other victims would still remain waiting and waiting.

I was waiting for my fate to take the final twist. Reluctantly, I found myself in another Hellish nightmare which led me to the end of this voyage. All these events in my life brought me the realisation that the paths of our souls are utterly mysterious and it takes more than one lifetime to understand the reason behind circumstances. At times we do not understand that these truths are beyond our grasp of facts.

It was so in my case. The sheer truth of my reality confronted me again, piercing my heart like blades. Another night came, which was similar to the other and what I did was the outcome, the release of many suppressed emotions of hatred which I buried deep within me. Then it was time for them to emerge. Yes, I've been compelled to do it and an inner force inside me propelled me to put an end to it, to violence.

It was a phone call which initiated, this step which ultimately led to my final destination. That afternoon Erika, who was still active in the team, called me one evening whilst I was at home.
Erika asked me to accompany her to a place where a woman had called her asking for help. I accepted and she came for me. Looking back, I wish it had not happened, for what followed was weaved on threads of oppression which led to my destruction. Yet, it was meant to be, for it put this entire saga to an end. That evening Erika was leading me to Hell. But then there was light.

It was almost evening when we arrived at our destination. The house we were visiting was rather large, situated in the country side. It was isolated, yet, overpowering and the people who lived there must have been very rich.

Erika rang the bell and a woman in her forties came to open and greeted us.
'Come in,' she said and we were led in.

SHATTERED WINGS

I could not help looking at her face, which was all bruised, even though she was wearing dark glasses to conceal her scars. Apart from her bruises, I noticed that her face was familiar. This was not the first time I have met this woman but I could not recall.

She asked us to sit down and we obeyed her.

'I've had enough now,' she started by saying, 'Look at me closely.'

Then she took off her glasses and I was horrified to see her eyes completely covered with bruises whilst her face was all scarred.

She continued, 'This is the result of my experience, but tell me, is rape considered in marriage?'

Erika looked at me and then said, 'Of course, rape is any act against a women's consent and even in the case of a married women. A woman has a right to be respected even in the framework of marriage.'

This woman was not only raped, but also physically abused and looking at her and listening to her filled me with rage. How far these men can go? When it comes to financial situation the woman lacked nothing, but was afflicted with violence, which made her appear equal with other women in her situation who are overshadowed by violence. There was no class, no age, for everyone was a subject to violence. This poor woman lowered her head and fiddled with her hands and then she put the glasses on and looked up at us.

'My name is Joan and this has been going on for years, but I had no courage to speak.'

She paused; her lips were forming into words again.

'I read about your centre and I decided to stop this lie, my husband has been violating me for these last ten years. He beats me, forces me to have sex, whenever he wants. Well, at first I accepted this situation, as I believed that it's a woman's duty to obey her husband. Also, he gives no option; he even threatens to kill me. One night he even violated me in front of my son.'

My God! I thought. What savage.
Joan hid her face between her hands and sobbed. Erica gripped her hand firmly and asked her in a low voice, 'Have you ever tried to discuss matters with him?'
Joan looked at Erika again, 'No miss. My husband is a sadist, I can't even talk with him, but when in public he is different and people do not believe me when I tell them. So, the best way was to remain silent.'
'And keep suffering,' Erika interrupted, 'And what does your husband do?' She asked her again.
'My husband is in politics, a member of Parliament.'

Her words struck me like thunder. A shiver ran all over my spine. The word politician echoed in my ear like thunder. I thought of the other one whose shadow I could not conceal from my memories. Then, I gazed at her, scrutinising her, trying to make the association. My God! It all came back now and the sudden realisation dawned upon me, leaving me breathless and I jolted from my seat. Yes, I knew her. Of, course she was familiar and this instant of recognition made me shudder and it would have been better for me if I had remained at home. I recalled those gloomy moments in hospital and now all the scenes appeared before me. In the scene, I pictured the last moments of the poor young boy in his last moments. I recalled his mother's face. She looked different then, a beautiful woman who lacked nothing yet, beneath her immaculate skin she was masking the deep shadows of violence which were her actual reality. This was the same violence which followed my steps.

Joan was Juan's mother and also the wife of that bastard. She was George's wife and no wonder he was violent to her, but in that moment my detestation for him increased. But what was I doing here, sitting in the lion's den.

No, this was not real, but a bad dream, because if it was reality, then life was a cruel jester, and I was its victim.

It was not a dream, and sitting there was like being taken in a voyage across time. Blades pierced my heart and I felt this reality suffocating me. Suddenly, I thought I was sensing his breath all over my body and I could even feel his footsteps approaching me and slowly, slowly he planned to grab me.

Now the room and everything in the house made me feel ill at ease. I could not stay here in the monster's property. I felt a complete stranger, an intruder and this was no longer my place. Whilst, Erika was listening emphatically to Joan, I plucked up my courage and moved quietly from the seat and headed for the doorway.

A feeling of relief swept all over me and the fresh air of the country side was blowing fiercely on my cheeks helped to alleviate my burdens. I was free at last, free from the recent news which was choking me. My feet took me away from his place and it felt good for a while. This was only for a while, but even now fate had made up its mind to taunt me again and this time with grave consequences.

Suddenly, I felt like choking again. Was it the wind blowing faster? Or my throat releasing itself. I had been wrong. No, it was not the wind nor the release, but the capturing hands of a monster who grabbed me. I felt a pair of hands suffocating me, and then I was released and felt myself being carried away to somewhere which was unfamiliar. I felt like being carried with the waves, but the strong arms were hurting me now and I tried to resist, to release myself, but the wind was against me.

I found myself in a car. This experience was not new to me, but with the sounds of the wind in my ears it took long to realise where I was heading to. At once, my eyes were opened to the reality which was facing me and it did not take me long to recognise the face of the monster whose devious act had overshadowed my life. Something warned me; this time there was no escape. I felt it like the blood pumping strongly in my veins.

This was not a dream, but the cruel claws of fate and after all that I've been through I was back again, unexpectedly back where I never dreamt to be. That was crossing his path again.

I recognised his voice and I heard him say, 'What the Hell are you doing here,'

What was I doing here? I did not even know what I had been doing here, but I knew that I wanted to escape from this place, most of all from him.

The courage came again, and I heard myself saying, 'George, leave me once and for all.'

'No Francine, I will not leave you,' he uttered with a harsh voice.

His arms were around my throat now and he was pressing hard, so hard that I could not breathe.

'I want to destroy you.'

I shivered as his breath and his words repulsed me. George was here again and there was no way out.

The bastard was going to kill me and this time he would succeed.

He then released me and started to drive the car, 'Let me go George,' I cried.

He smiled sardonically, 'No, I will not let you go, you are my hostage.'

George burst out laughing and his laughing hammered in my ears, making me feel uneasy. This time there was no escape from him and the best way was to surrender.

All was over for me and the only path which followed was death. I thought of Erika, she must be missing me by now, but I was lost to her, and lost to the centre. And there was more to come.

This was far worse than the first incident. George stopped his car, but I had no idea where I. From what I could see, this was a remote place which was rather new to me and being alone in this place, now I knew what to expect and the tragedy which befall upon me was that I could do nothing and hope has forsaken me and left me buried in the dark.

The time has come for the descending of my soul in the deepest abyss of the Hell. Now, George came closer, so close that I could feel his breath, which took me again to the dark shadow. It was going to happen again, with the difference that I had been prepared for the next station as my feet had already walked on this territory. Now, my heart was turned to stone and nothing now could melt the strong ice which surmounted every corner of my heart.

His lips were coming close to mine. Suddenly, as if to taunt me, the image of Gino appeared before my eyes. He was lost in the desert of eternity, but I longed for his lips now which were now fierce and cruel, ready to take away what was left of me. But what was left of me?

George was kissing me hard on my lips, I tried to move away, but I knew that there was no escape now that he was lost in passion

He stopped abruptly.

SHATTERED WINGS

'Leave me, George,' I uttered firmly.
'No is a yes, your body wants me and mine wants you, I am dying to taste you again.'
His cruel words sank deep inside me. That was all, the carnal lust which constrained him to resort to violence, to rape and ardent greed.

I made an effort to leave the car, but he knew how to play his cards well, the car was locked and I was locked endorsed with this dark shadow.
'George, why don't you leave me alone? Is it not enough what you did to me that night, you raped me, and made me kill my child, your seed inside me. I have become a murderess, because of you.'

I stopped and he was staring at me, watching me intently almost disbelieving my words. These words were my only triumph over him and I took opportunity of it. This was my revenge on him to hurt his ego. For some men, each abortion is the killing of their son. He is the man and I killed his male ego, the seed which could have become another man. A wave of satisfaction was incited deep within me, for certainly he would be hurt with these words after losing a child. At that moment I wanted him to suffer like I did many years before, but I doubted it with a man so callous.

He had to say something to save his pride for he said, 'You could have told me. That would have changed everything between us my dear,' he said giggling.
'Did you expect me to tell you?' I yelled. 'But I have no regrets in destroying your bastard'

Following these words, anything could happen, but there was nothing to lose, my soul was already lost. It did not matter now if the hysteric demon inside him took over me. I have provoked it and now, with courage, I waited for his reaction. What mattered was that he felt injured and dejected the same feelings which he instigated in my life. Because of him I could not love other men, because of him the woman inside me became a murderer, killing my own womanhood. It was all over and soon I was going to fade with the wind.

Yet, the tears were rolling faster now on my cheeks, as if betraying my heart which wanted to remain intact and hard. It was torn into pieces. I buried my face in both hands and cried. But why? Even death was deserting me now?

Just when I needed it.

His response was laughter and he laughed in my face and I heard him say again.
'My dear, then I will give you another one.'
Shameful brute! I thought. This dirty man was a politician and dared to appear in public. Who will be there to unravel his sins? But, if I had any regrets for removing my child, now there was none. My actions were now justified when confronted with this bastard and this led me to complete freedom. But I was not free from him yet. Not yet. He has come again to haunt me, persecute and relive my memory of his forced violence. Had I really forgotten it? No, but now it was being vividly

brought back to my memory and I knew it was going to happen again.

He was speaking again, 'You're a child Francine, you were on the papers and set up that centre, what did you think? That you were going to stop men's lust? You'd have to be a man to understand what a man feels inside his pants.'

His words were making me sick, but I could not escape, locked in the car with him. There was only space for the manifestation of passion and violence which regained his ego again. The shadow of rape was peering at me, what was next where the boundaries of my body were going to be invaded again.

He was speaking again, 'You are created for us, to satisfy our passions, our force or no. Francine, you are a slut, like all woman and you're mine.'

His words angered me and I could not control myself. I slapped on his right cheek.

'You have respect, not even for yourself.'

'We are the rulers and no whore can defy us. You cannot out number us.'

He touched his cheeks and smiled as to defy me.

His words made me furious. Suddenly panic seized me and I put my hands around his neck and attempted to smother him, but he was stronger than me and removed my hands away from his throat. This added to my frustration and now I could do nothing and then I spat at on his face.

George burst out laughing and behind that hilarious laughter I could feel he was he was contriving something.

My battle was lost.

His thin filthy lips were forming into words now.
'Francine, I pity you. If only you listened to me, but you were stubborn. You wanted to go deeper and thought you could stop us with your center. After all, women want to be violated. That was why they came to our centre. '
He was laughing again and I could not bear him any longer.
'And now my princess, my woeful lover you know the secret.'
'You are crazy!' I yelled.
'No, my dear. Now you must die for knowing our secret.'
Despair overwhelmed me, but there was no time and I had no way out.

Then his hard hands played with my hair and then his hands moved to my blouse. I was expecting this and I only prayed that this would be fast. Like a violent beast he brought his lips closer to mine. His breath was horrible and his mouth felt like glue. The monster's hands tore my blouse and searched for my breasts, and then all his body was all over me, to the extent that I could not release myself. Like he did before and now it was easy for him. I cried, but no one could hear my cry, not even the wind. His body felt heavy on mine and then with his hands he tore my skirt and headed for my underpants, invading my intimate territories.

His breath smelt pungent. With my eyes closed I felt him entering deep inside me, and the pain came back and it went deeper. I could not utter any single word, as if words have completely vanished from my throat. Now every movement of this meant more pain and inner spasms.
He was inside me again and the monster was invading me, hurting the wound between my thighs.

It did not matter now, as I knew the feeling and I could endure it. For Francine it was over and fate had carried her again to the depths of abyss. I felt lost again and my spirit was invaded and this time there was no return. For, yes, indeed rape is an invasion of soul, of the mind of all and the only escape was the division between the two women.

It seemed that both of them wanted to leave.

There were no stars to look at me, to console me and soothe my pain. I was alone with the dark clouds and encircled by his fluids. George had won again and tonight he would celebrate his manhood, his male ego.

With my eyes closed I waited for death, but death did not come, another shadow which deceived me. Instead there was this monster panting inside and I couldn't resist. An inner voice whispered in my ears. Do not let him win.

No, I could not let him win. I will die, but he will too.

When all was over he looked at me and he was going to say something.
'Do you love me?' he asked with an ironic tone in his voice.
Love him? I could love no man. They were all bastards, but his voice brought me back to reality. I was there in his car, facing this beast. I despised him, 'No George.' I shouted at him, 'I abhor you, now go to Hell.'

A sudden force came over me. I hit him, scratched his face, but it was all in vain. Instead he was laughing heartily, 'You know you look beautiful even when you say you hate me. You turn me on.'
Then it was it. My eyes fell on an iron poker on the back seat. With all my effort I forced my hands to the back seat and grabbed it. With the poker in my hands I felt a new overwhelming force compelling me to act. Then I did it. Yes, all my hatred my hands picked up the iron poker and a wave of energy passed from my heart to my hands.

I hit him with the poker, right on his head. He moaned with pain and with his left hand he pulled my hair with all his remaining strength. He was hurting me, but it was not for long for he suddenly withdrew back. Then I saw blood all over the car, his body was covered with blood and he laid motionless. His face looked ghastly pale and his eyes stared lifeless.

I also remained motionless, staring at him. I had killed him.

Murderess, an inner voice admonished me, for the second time. My heart pounded. He was dead and I did not know whether to cry or smile. I've had my revenge, but the coldness of death was overwhelming me. Panic seized me. I touched his hands and face to reassure myself that he was gone. My body shivered and I wanted to get away. I looked at my hands, clammy and stained with his blood. What could I do? I was still locked with him in his car.

Will I die with him? No, not here, it will be somewhere else. I was already dead. Francine was only a walking spirit, was I? My eyes fell again on the poker and I gripped it and I hit the door. The glass fell into pieces, another hit, another one, and finally the door was opened.

I managed to get out, but a part of me was still locked inside. My body shivered, but I walked away from the car, away from the beast, yet, his marks inflated me, his ardent breath permeated my soul. I kept walking, feeling the soft breezing caressing my half naked body. Little did it matter now; I was already used to this nakedness, the loss of dignity stinging beneath my skin. Their shadows were walking with me as well, engraved on my hands.

The Angel of Death! I thought. Where was he?

Tears streamed all over my face. Why all this? And I asked again, why do men rape? No answer, but my feet kept throbbing on small rocks which were hurting and burning my feet. Tonight I was meeting him, him whom I encountered everyday in my work.

I thought of Erika, the centre, the victims, who like me had been drifted in this Hell. Yet, they stood there remained in my past and I had no right to go back. Murderess, the voices cried within me. Then I heard the child crying and crying. 'You're a murderess,' I heard them say in my inner ears, 'You must die.'

My feet walked and walked, until I headed to the edge of the cliffs. Yes, this time I had to go and I will succeed. My feet were relieved from the pain and hard rubbing of the ground and the waves were waiting for Francine, the murderess who took the life of an important man and his child.
Then I saw the little girl with black hair and big dark eyes. She was looking at me, watching me intently and then she smiled. I saw her dancing around and then came back, transformed into a young woman and her lips were soft and ripe dreaming of their first kiss.

Innocent velvet, stained with the kiss of blood.

She was raped, killed. Again, I saw her smiling and her eyes were shining as she walked in the dull long corridors of hospital. 'He is here,' she whispered.
'Who?'

SHATTERED WINGS

Then I saw him. Ivan was there at the edge of the cliffs. He was the same, but his hair was grey and vague.

'Ivan,' I cried, 'why, did you betray me? Ivan, if you loved me all this would be changed.'

'But I love you,' he said. Then he disappeared as well with my life.

Ivan's image faded and the little girl appeared again.

'Francine,' she whispered, 'Francine,' she repeated. I felt myself swaying and falling on the ground. The faint light of dawn was disturbing me, bringing me back to this reality, opening my eyes. I found myself lying on the ground. Where was I? Was this the next dimension? Then I recognised the surroundings.

No, I was still on earth and had a bad dream. But my clothes, my hands were stained with blood. 'What happened?' I asked myself. It all came before me like a sequence a murder in a film, there had been a murder and I was the author of all.

I trembled and a feeling of apprehension over powered me. My God! I pictured all the media talking about him. And I was the criminal, not the victim.

I thought of my family, my friends, of Erika. All was lost, I have failed, deceived my fate. Silence stood on the horizon and only the sun was rising at the surface.

It was giving birth to a new day. Birth! How could I talk of birth when I had been the creator of death? I was a direct collaborator with him, the Angel of Death.

George was going to remain stained in the palms of my hands. There was a new day and I had no alternative now but to go back with the flow.

Going with the flow meant my feet leading me to the village, to the first police station. I had to pay for killing a man, above all, an important man on the island, who deserved respect. But did he not commit murder before that night he raped a young woman who had not yet seen the sun rising on her rounded breasts and its reflection in her inner velvet.

SHATTERED WINGS

DOCTOR MICHELLE

Francine's ordeal left me speechless. I was dumbfounded by her story. This young woman, sitting before me, was devastated and torn into pieces caused by rape. Rape is the masterpiece of my patients, the ones who bluntly and, with not any slightest emotion, retell their stories as if nothing was wrong.

And what about their victims? They carry the seeds buried inside them for years. Both stood at the far end, yet, I could not but feel admiration for this lovely woman. Her big eyes were watching intently.

'So what's going to happen now?' she asked.
'I will present a report in court.'
She lowered her head and looked confused, then looked at me again.
'He was very important and the court will be on his side.'
I held her hands firmly, 'No Justice sees the case through objective eyes,' I added.
'But please take me out of here. All these walls are reminding me of him.'
'I know,' I said tenderly.
'No,' she answered in a loud voice, 'Sorry, but you can never understand because you didn't go through it. Rape will remain with me throbbing in my veins. In my memories there is always him, penetrating me, all the time.'

Francine covered her face with both hands. At that moment I was touched, but as a professional that I was, I managed to control myself.

For an instant, Jimmy came into my mind and I thought of him and of the way he raped girls. I could picture him clearly raping the girls who are now prisoners to his lust. Like Francine, locked in a prison but buried in another one, that was her past, where her perpetrator controlled every breath of her life.

All I could do was to promise to help her, to finish the report as soon as I could. This entailed a lot of work.

Back home I kept thinking of Francine and her case. This woman instilled in me new hope and brought me face to face with the reality of rape and sexual offences. For most of the time I looked at my clients as people whom I had to control. I listened to their stories, yet had little space for the victims.

Rape is defined as sexual intercourse or penetration without the consent of the victim. There are other jurisdictions which define rape, not only by the penetration of the male sexual organ, but any other objects such as finger or objects. However, I was not going to debate about this, as whatever case, it is still without the person's consent. A person said no and should be respected. This, at times, is an issue which my patients do not understand, or better they were not brought up to take no for an answer. And going back to my court report, I wonder who was the criminal, Francine or her perpetrator. Whatever rape is a reality which often is hidden, turned in silence, the sufferings, the agonies are endless and most women do not report to the police in fear of what might happen afterwards.

Francine's case illustrates this, and I believe that she should have proceeded with the case and that brings me to the topic of giving more help to rape victims. The victims should report immediately and should be given information about how to cultivate the evidence which can be used later in court. After the incidence of rape victims go through shock and feel adrift in a world which no longer pertain them. The victims feel dirty and the first reaction would be to withdraw and go and wash themselves.

This will completely eradicate the presence of certain evidence which will then be used in court to prove the perpetrator's guilt. These include pubic hair of the aggressor, and traces of sperm and also injuries inflicted on the victim.

It is of utmost importance for the victim to seek immediate help from friends, relatives and professionals who will then support her and take her to the police. The victim should be given support while she is giving her evidence to the police and throughout the whole procedures. Most victims do not report the crime of rape in fear and lack of information of the procedures followed after rape such as the police, the medical examination and the court. By doing so they are giving power to the aggressor in harming another victim. Most likely they do so. It is no use debating on how and why it happened. Victims should never take the blame for the perpetrator's actions. It has nothing to do with the way she was dressed or behaved, but rather a subjective feeling of an individual who could not control his impulses.

The effects of rape create intense emotions, where the victim may have constant memories and nightmares. Victims find it hard to concentrate, sleep, eat and to function normally. These symptoms result in Acute Stress Disorder and the symptoms are numerous, most of the time the victims will feel strange and find it hard to remember part of the assault. For instance, the victim seeks to avoid the places and feelings which remind her of the assault.

Initially, after the assault, the victim goes through emotional shock. She feels numb and shows no emotion. This is a natural defense mechanism to protect her from severe stress. Often, she asks, did it really happen? Here, the victim goes through the phase of disbelief, where she knows that something has happened to her, but cannot register it as if it was not happening to her. Fear is what follows and the victim may fear that the rapist will threaten her or that she will not be believed. Also, the fear of getting pregnant or contracting a sexually transmitted disease.

Another thing which embarrasses the victim is talking about rape. This may be shameful for a victim who has gone through the experience of rape and describing step by step in precise detail on what happened to other professionals, the police and courts creates a feeling of shame and embarrassment.

In most cases, survivors of rape tend to feel guilty, as if they have promulgated the rape. They feel that they provoked the rape or that they could have done something to prevent it.   Shame and the feeling of dirt is not uncommon, the victim feels invaded in a harsh, unwanted way and seeks way to eliminate this intrusion. This is often done by taking showers regularly, hoping to get rid of the memory or far worse the shadow of the rapists. And this is where anger and rage directed at their attacker and even at life emerges.

This symptoms are defined Rape Trauma Syndrome, which are the effects which follow after the rape. Many women respond differently from each other. There are many effects which are physical, emotional and psychological and these depend only on the circumstances surrounding the victim. Rape Trauma Syndrome comes into two stages, which is the Acute Phase and the long term.

Through the immediate phase, the victim responds emotionally into what is called expressed emotions and controlled emotions. The expressed emotions are fear, anger and anxiety and controlled emotions include shock and numbness which conceal the victim's feelings after the assault.

There are also physical reactions, such as lack of sleep, nightmares, and changes in the way of eating, like increased appetite or lack of it, pain in the stomach. Throughout this phase the victim goes through mood swings. She can go through the assault again, trying to figure out what really happened or she can block it completely from their memory, persuading herself that it did not happen. The common feelings are fear, anger, embarrassment, shame and revenge.

In the long term phase, the victim seeks to change her life completely and this is an attempt to gain control over her life again. She may change her residence, her appearance, go to self defense classes and introduce anything which makes her feel safe again. Fear does not leave either, and the victim most often experiences fear of being alone, of having sex, or of being with other people. Often, the nightmares and dreams return again, where the victim dreams of being in the scene of rape. By time and healing they will ebb away. This is a process which takes time and support is very important at this stage and it helps to facilitate healing. Other victims are not as lucky as their other sisters. There were victims who suffered permanent disabilities and even dead.

Pregnancy following rape is rare, but when it occurs it will create inner conflicts and add to the trauma of rape. One would debate the woman may be infertile in the time she was raped or that the trauma itself might inhibit ovulation. Yet, though rare there were cases and women who resorted to abortion cannot be judged or condemned. It may be the easiest solution, but it has long term effects. The question will always be whether to keep the child or not. In other cases, victims chose to give their child away for adoption for they could not bear to think of the child. It will always remind them of their trauma. The other option would be emergency contraception, more known as the morning after pill. This is a high dosage of birth control and is recommended after sexual assault over a period of seventy two hours. Some pro life groups consider this to be abortive and this opens room for discussion.

I detest thinking again of violence against women in armed conflicts. Rape is not by chance but has its purpose that to be used as a military objective. These objectives may be ethnic cleansing, to create political terror, to obtain information and as a reward to soldiers. Women are always a target for violence and suffer deeply. Rape is against the Geneva Convention but still continues to be used. This takes me again to the Second World War, where Nazi soldiers raped women in the Soviet Union and in revenge the Soviets, more known as the Red Army, created mass rape of German women, one town after the other.

Every woman in Berlin, regardless of age or beauty, was a fair game for the revengeful soldiers. Unfortunately, man does not learn and wars are repeated. Rape remains part of this game. The contempt of one nation for the other was projected in sexual violence.

Here, I think of the case of conflicts in Bosnia, former Yugoslavia. In 1992 Bosnian women were detained by Bosnian Serb Forces and were raped repeatedly. Erika's recounting experience gives a detailed explanation of what happened in Bosnia, the so called ethnic cleansing of rape camps. The Serbs built up rape camps which were targeted to rape women. Croatians, Bosnian Muslims and even Catholics were amongst the victims, ages ranged from six years old and eighty year old women. I shudder when I think of the girls, the same girls who were raped by my patients. These women were raped in the presence of their families and forced to leave their homes. Some of them never returned. Others got pregnant and had to seek abortion and psychiatric help. Rape was a tool to inflict fear and terror in bringing people out of the country.

It also served to boost men's morale. Fortunately, proceedings have been undertaken in the International Courts and this gave victims the opportunity to proceed against their attackers. The International Criminal Tribunal was established in February 1993 by the United Nations Security Council. This court was the first international war crimes court since the Nuremberg trials following the second World war.

Yet, rape prevailed even in recent wars and I was appalled to read about rape of Iraqi women in the early days of US occupation. There were numerous reports of sexual violence reported by Iraqi girls and women. These facts are repulsive and shocking, but devastatingly real.

*

No, matter how hard we endear to omit them, they come back to haunt us like patients.
They were no different, but they premeditated or were propelled to abuse their victims. Nevertheless, the acts are the same with the same effects on their victims.

With painstaking precision and hard work, my report was finalised. I have to admit, it was not an easy task, but with attention and a little help from God I arrived to my conclusions. I presented the report, and my conclusions were that Francine had no psychiatric problems, but suffered from trauma after having to go through rape again.

Later, Francine was not found guilty and was thus set free. A beautiful day dawned, with the sun bestowing its rays on this woman of iron. It turned out that George formed part of a secret society that derived sexual satisfaction by raping young woman. This was also described by Jennifer, who joined the centre and that was one reason why the centre had been burnt and destroyed.

A better day dawned for Erika and other victims who suffered in silence. Francine taught me a lesson and in her beautiful eyes I saw not only courage, but the real façade of rape and sexual aggression.

In my profession I only come face to face with the other aspect and like Francine I put the same question. What about the men who rape? Will they ever stop? I can't find the answer, no, not in their cold eyes and hard hearts. They will not control the sexual urges which compel them to rape an innocent girl or angel. Controlling sex offenders may raise a never ending debate, but victims and the community need to be protected. These patients are most likely to be recidivists, and they are arrested and convicted for the same offences. Some of the risks are when the offender has little or no support system.

The offender thinks he is entitled to sex. If he the offender has access to potential victims and if the offender is hostile and angry, or abusing drugs and alcohol. If the offender persistently denies his involvement and keep blaming the victim for the crime.

Given the rates of recidivism gathered from arrest, conviction and incarceration and the repetition of crime, it is our duty to protect victims. My conclusions may be that we are spending money to lock these people up, restraining them for a period of time, yet at the same time we are given no guarantee that they will not re-offend. I once read that there were prisoners in some states who asked to be chemically castrated, as they were certain that they were going to do it again. This brings me to the notion that prison only constraints them for a while, but then what?

Then we get their answers, more far worse their victims.

Another form of control is the sex offenders tracking, where persons who were convicted of specified sex crimes are required to register within the local law enforcement. Sex offenders are expected to update their personal information regularly. This serves as a form of control, at least to track them.

We can reduce sexual abuse through treatment, where it can be combined with other criminal justice responsibilities such as probation, incarceration and community supervision. Medical treatment and Psychotherapy are what work, where treatment enables offenders to understand their actions and learn to take responsibility for their actions. It instills motivation in them and helps them to change their harmful conduct. With training, offenders learn to identify the chain of thoughts and motives that could lead to a sexual offence.

Treatment has to be continuous and if necessary throughout their lives, permanently. Yet, once they have served their prison sentence or supervision order, most perpetrators are free, free to rape again. Most of them stop the treatment the day after and then we get them back in prison or in hospital.

Our clients are tough, and a big headache in the justice system. Well, laws and policies have to be emended or introduced to facilitate this. If not, we will keep having them raping us women, men and our children.

Can we afford to create victims? Of course, not.

Perhaps both of them are victims. One day they could have been innocent children who were introduced to sexual abuse, but we cannot keep on paying their price. And I ask myself again; Is this enough? I recall the sessions with my patients and their looks piercing like daggers, hard looks peering at me, looking far at their victims. Will their inner urges stop one day?

Silence reigns on the desk where the files are standing, one on the other. Each file retells a story, each report tells of a new nightmare for a girl or women.

And I still think of Joseph s' words ...
'I felt I was living again. Yes, I am a rapist and no one can stop me. No court, no law can refrain my passions. I may stop for a while, but then I go back to my dream. You still have to find ways to stop me from dreaming. Until then I will keep on raping if not in reality, certainly in my dreams.'

On my desk there is new addition, another file, that of Francine. It is closed, but her story remains forever engraved in my memory. For Francine and Erika I will use pain, misfortune to create new light. My light lies in preventing them from re-offending and that would be control and treatment.

Treatment permanently!

Will it be real, or a wishful thinking idea of a psychiatrist who carries the burden of working every day with devastation created by violent behaviour?

FRANCINE

Without any doubt, my case created immense speculation. George was a Member of Parliament and when the truth came out there was a scandal, but there were other people who showed solidarity with my case and supported me.

Dr Michelle was very helpful, not only did she help me in court, but offered continuous support to me and my family. It was all over. My journey had to stop here, yet I was not the same anymore. This journey left its mark on my soul, but it was not all in vain, I had survived, surmounted the threads of pain and desperation.

After the tempest the sun came out. It came out for me as well.

There were two messages awaiting me. The first one was not so good. It was a letter from Salvatore. It had been like ages yet my heart still fluttered and echoed like drums in the desert. The letter brought bad news, which left me stunned. Ivan was dead. He died in a car accident, on exactly the same night of my tragedy. I marveled at the contrasting synchronicity between these two men. Both of them left that night. This sent shivers all over my spine. So it was really him, Ivan, the one I saw on the cliffs. Strange, yet interesting how these two men, very different from one another, had managed to deceive me in ways which left me bereft and devastated; shattered but not for long.

SHATTERED WINGS

Yes, maybe with Ivan it was different. There was no anger in my heart, but compassion, perhaps I still loved him.

For George there was only spite and contempt.

Life had to go on. The second piece of news was much better. This time it was from Erika, my soul companion. She brought me the news, as it was she who gave birth to the idea. The centre was going to be built again and this time nothing would stop us. Now, I knew who was behind the threat, the stalking, and finally the burning of the centre. He was no longer on this earth.

A chapter in my life is closed now.

Tonight, while I am writing the last notes of my record, I look at the moon. She is glowing in her full gown, casting her light, perhaps even protecting us from the lust of men.

But, it occurs to me that this night, this hour, could bring new pain for another victim. I pray for them without forgetting the one who is creating violence. If only he could see the same light of the Goddess Moon. That would perhaps decrease his sufferings and on others.

They say that forgiveness is the light which leads us to our healing. It's not that easy. Even now, while I am setting my story on paper, there is another woman who is burying another story deep within her. My only consolation is the moon, and to her I put my prayers, my dreams. What can we do to stop men from raping? There is no answer, but in compensation the moon offers her peace, and my heart is opened again.

Almost six months elapsed from my trial and everything was falling into place. One fine day, I decided to visit the temples, to share with them my dawn of healing. The temples remained there, intact and silent, sharing my grief. It was the 21st June, the day which marked the Equinox and the beginning of summer.

Indeed, there was a new summer awaiting me. Whilst I was lost admiring these huge spirits, hoping to travel in their immensity, a familiar voice brought me back to reality.
'Francine,' said the voice.
I looked back and was astounded but happy. Gino was standing beside me.
He then took my hands and kissed it.
'Gino, I am sorry,' I heard myself saying.
'Francine, I know everything and I am ready to take the journey with you.'
I stopped pondering. Of, course; he heard it in the news. Then I looked into his eyes and they were different from the others. In his gaze there was no lust like George, and no seeds of betrayal like those incited by Ivan. His eyes promised truth. I looked at the temples and they stood motionless, but approving. Then I kissed him on his lips and a wave of heat showed me that I could start the journey.

SHATTERED WINGS

So, today I am still following this path, yet I still dream of a world where men do not use violence, and I will not give up the fight to control their urges. Time will pass, as it has done for centuries, and time has the power to heal. Perhaps it has, for a while. A woman, who has been raped, invaded by the power of violence, will never forget that day.

Even if fate smiles again, there within her lies the fear, the apprehension that it might happen again to her. This is a shadow which walks continuously with my soul.

I will never forget, it fades for a while, but it comes back. Yet still I win. Do I forgive? This is an answer which my soul cannot give. Perhaps, I will try one day, but when I think of it, the shadows of darkness overtake me and fill me with consternation.

So I would rather end here and close the chapter of my story and that is where another journey begins.

That is my journey against rape.

If only this word could be cancelled forever from our planet! That is another dream, but at least different and I dream it in every hour of the day.